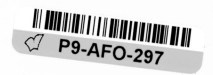
P9-AFO-297

Programming

and

Metaprogramming

in

The Human Biocomputer

PROGRAMMING AND METAPROGRAMMING

IN THE HUMAN BIOCOMPUTER

THEORY AND EXPERIMENTS

JOHN C. LILLY, M.D.

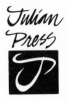

Based on a series of seminars given at the Department of Psychiatry, Schools of Medicine, Johns Hopkins University, University of California at Los Angeles, University of Minnesota; at the Medical Seminar, Edgewood Arsenal; and at the Conference of Science, Philosophy and Religion, Jewish Theological Seminary, New York, in 1966.

Copyright © 1967, 1968 by John C. Lilly, M.D.

All rights reserved. No part of this book may be reproduced or transmitted
in any form or by any means, electronic or mechanical, including photocopying,
recording, or by any information storage and retrieval system,
without permission in writing from the publisher.

Published by The Julian Press, Inc., a member of the Crown Publishing Group,
distributed by Crown Publishers, Inc., 225 Park Avenue South, New York,
New York 10003 and represented in Canada by the Canadian MANDA Group

Julian Press and colophon are trademarks of The Julian Press, Inc.

Manufactured in the United States of America

Library of Congress Catalog Card Number 72-189950

ISBN 0-517-52757-X
10 9 8 7 6 5 4 3 2 1
1987 Edition

□ Contents

List of Figures

List of Tables

¤ Author's Note

This work has a curious history. It was written as a final summary report to a government agency (National Institute of Mental Health) concerning five years of my life work. (The agency paid my salary for the five years.)

It was conceived from a space rarer these days than it was then: the laws suspending scientific interest, research, involvement and decisions about d-lysergic acid di-ethyl amide tartate were passed just as this particular work was completed; the researchers were inadequately consulted (put down, in fact). The legislators composed laws in an atmosphere of desperation. The national negative program on LSD was launched; LSD was the big scare, on a par with War, Pestilence, and Famine as the destroyer of young brains, minds and fetuses.

In this atmosphere (1966-1967) *Programming and Metaprogramming in The Human Biocomputer* was written. The work and its notes are dated from 1964 to 1966. The conception was formed in 1949, when I was first exposed to computer design ideas by Britton Chance. I coupled these ideas back to my own software through the atmosphere of my neurophysiological research on cerebral cortex. It was more fully elaborated in the tank isolation solitude and confinement work at NIMH from 1953 to 1958, run in parallel with the neurophysiological research on the rewarding and punishing systems in the brain. The dolphin research was similarly born in the tank, with brain electrode results as parents in the further conceptions.

While I was writing this work, I was a bit too fearful to express candidly in writing the direct experience, uninterpreted. I felt that a group of thirty persons' salaries, a large research budget, a whole Institute's life depended on me and what I wrote. If I wrote the data up straight, I would have rocked the boats of several lives (colleagues and family) beyond my own stabilizer effectiveness threshold, I hypothesized.

Despite my precautionary attitude, the circulation in 1967 of this work contributed to the withdrawal of research funds in 1968 from the research program on dolphins by one government agency. I heard several negative stories regarding my brain and mind, altered by LSD. At this point I closed the Institute and went to the Maryland Psychiatric Research Center to resume LSD research under government auspices. I introduced the ideas in work to the MPRC researchers and I left for the Esalen Institute in 1969.

At Esalen my involvement in direct human gut-to-gut communication and lack of involvement in administrative responsibility brought my courage to the sticking place. Meanwhile, Stewart Brand of the Whole Earth Truck Catalog (Menlo Park, Calif.) reviewed the work in the Whole Earth Catalog from a mimeographed copy I had given W. W. Harmon of Stanford for his Sufic purposes. Stewart wrote me asking for copies to sell. I had 300 printed photo-offset from the typed copy. He sold them in a few weeks and asked permission to reprint on newsprint an enlarged version at a lower price. Sceptical about salability, I agreed. Book People, Berkeley, arranged the reprinting. Several thousand copies were sold.

I had written the report in such a way that its basic messages were hidden behind a heavy long introduction designed to stop the usual reader. Apparently once word got out, this device no longer stalled the interested readers. Somehow the basic messages were important enough to enough readers so that the work acquired an unexpected viability. Thus it seems appropriate to reprint it in full.

On several different occasions, I have been asked to rewrite this work. One such start at rewrite ended up as another book. (*The Center of the Cyclone*, The Julian Press, Inc., New York, 1972.) Another start is evolving into my book number five (*Simulations of God: A Science of Belief*). It seems as if this older work is a seminating source for other works and solidly resists revision. To me it is a thing separate from me, a record from a past space, a doorway into new spaces through which I passed and cannot return.

J.C.L.

February 1972
Los Angeles, California

¤ Preface to Second Edition [*]

All human beings, all persons who reach adulthood in the world today are programmed biocomputers. No one of us can escape our own nature as programmable entities. Literally, each of us may be our programs, nothing more, nothing less.

Despite the great varieties of programs available, most of us have a limited set of programs. Some of these are built-in. The structure of our nervous system reflects its origins in simpler forms of organisms from sessile protozoans, sponges, corals through sea worms, reptiles and proto-mammals to primates to apes to early anthropoids to humanoids to man. In the simpler basic forms, the programs were mostly built-in: from genetic codes to fully-formed organisms adultly reproducing, the patterns of function of action-reaction were determined by necessities of survival, of adaptation to slow environmental changes, of passing on the code to descendents.

As the size and complexity of the nervous system and its bodily carrier increased, new levels of programmability appeared, not tied to immediate survival and eventual reproduction. The built-in programs survived as a basic underlying context for the new levels, excitable and inhibitable, by the overlying control systems. Eventually, the cerebral cortex appeared as an expand-

---

*Quoted in entirety from John C. Lilly, *Simulations of God: A Science of Belief*, in preparation, 1972.

ing new high-level computer controlling the structurally lower levels of the nervous system, the lower built-in programs. For the first time learning and its faster adaptation to a rapidly changing environment began to appear. Further, as this new cortex expanded over several millions of years, a critical size of cortex was reached. At this new level of structure, a new capability emerged: learning to learn.

When one learns to learn, one is making models, using symbols, analogizing, making metaphors, in short, inventing and using language, mathematics, art, politics, business, etc. At the critical brain (cortex) size, languages and its consequences appear.

To avoid the necessity of repeating *learning to learn, symbols, metaphors, models* each time, I symbolize the underlying idea in these operations as *metaprogramming*. Metaprogramming appears at a critical cortical size — the cerebral computer must have a large enough number of interconnected circuits of sufficient quality for the operations of metaprogramming to exist in that biocomputer.

Essentially, metaprogramming is an operation in which a central control system controls hundreds of thousands of programs operating in parallel simultaneously. This operation in 1972 is not yet done in man-made computers — metaprogramming is done outside the big solid-state computers by the human programmers, or more properly, the human metaprogrammers. All choices and assignments of what the solid-state computers do, how they operate, what goes into them are still human biocomputer choices. Eventually, we may construct a metaprogramming computer, and turn these choices over to it.

When I said we may be our programs, nothing more, nothing less, I meant the substrate, the basic substratum under all else, of our metaprograms is our programs. All we are as humans is what is built-in and what has been acquired, and what we make of both of these. So we are one more result of the program substrate — the self-metaprogrammer.

As out of several hundreds of thousands of the substrate programs comes an adaptable changing set of thousands of metaprograms, so out of the metaprograms as substrate comes something else — the controller, the steersman, the programmer in the biocomputer, the self-metaprogrammer. In a well-organized biocomputer, there is at least one such critical control metaprogram labeled *I* for acting on other metaprograms and labeled *me* when acted upon by other metaprograms. I say *at least one* advisedly. Most of us have several controllers, selves, self-metaprograms which divide control among them, either in time parallel or in time series in sequences of control. As I will give in detail later, one path for *self-development* is to centralize control of one's biocomputer in one self-metaprogrammer, making the others into conscious executives subordinate to the single administrator, the single superconscient self-metaprogrammer. With appropriate methods, this centralizing of control, the elementary unification operation, is a realizable state for many, if not all biocomputers.

Beyond and above in the control hierarchy, the position of this single administrative self-metaprogrammer and his staff, there may be other controls and controllers, which, for convenience, I call **supraself metaprograms**. These are many or one depending on current states of consciousness in the single self-metaprogrammer. These may be personified *as if entities*, treated as if a network for information transfer, or *realized* as if self traveling in the Universe to strange lands or dimensions or spaces. If one does a further unification operation on these supraself metaprograms, one may arrive at a concept labeled *God, the Creator, the Starmaker,* or whatever. At times we are tempted to pull together apparently independent supraself sources *as if* one. I am not sure that we are quite ready to do this supraself unification operation and have the result correspond fully to an objective reality.

Certain states of consciousness result from and cause operation of this apparent unification phenomenon. We are still general purpose computers who can program any conceivable model of the universe inside our own structure, reduce the single self-metaprogrammer to a micro size, and program him to travel through his own model as if real (level 6, Satori +6: Lilly, 1972). This property is useful when one steps outside it and sees it for what it is — an immensely satisfying realization of the programmatic power of one's own biocomputer. To over-value or to negate such experiences is not a necessary operation. To realize that one has this property is an important addition to one's self-metaprogrammatic list of probables.

Once one has control over modelling the universe inside one's self, and is able to vary the parameters satisfactorily, one's self may reflect this ability by changing appropriately to match the new property.

The quality of one's model of the universe is measured by how well it matches the real universe. There is no guarantee that one's current model does match the reality, no matter how certain one feels about the high quality of the match. Feelings of awe, reverence, sacredness and certainty are also adaptable metaprograms, attachable to any model, not just the best fitting one.

Modern science knows this: we know that merely because a culture generated a cosmology of a certain kind and worshipped with it, was no guarantee of goodness of fit with the real universe. Insofar as they are testable, we now proceed to test (rather than to worship) models of the universe. Feelings such as awe and reverence are recognized as biocomputer energy sources rather than as determinants of truth, i.e., of the goodness of fit of models vs. realities. A pervasive feeling of certainty is recognized as a property of a state of consciousness, a special space, which may be indicative or suggestive but is no longer considered as a final judgement of a true fitting. Even as one can travel inside one's models inside one's head, so can one travel *outside* or be *the outside* of one's model of the universe, still inside one's head (see Lilly 1972: level or state +3, Satori +3). In this metaprogram it is as if one joins the creators, unites with God, etc. Here one can so attenuate the self that it may disappear.

One can conceive of other supraself metaprograms farther out than these, such as are given in Olaf Stapledon's *The Starmaker* (Dover, New York, 1937). Here the self joins other selves, touring the reaches of past and future time and of space, everywhere. The planet-wide consciousness joins into solar systems consciousness into galaxy-wide consciousness. Intergalactic sharing of consciousness fused into the mind of the universe finally faces its creator, the Starmaker. The universe's mind realizes that its creator knows its imperfections and will tear it down to start over, creating a more perfect universe.

Such uses of one's own biocomputer as the above can teach one profound truths about one's self, one's capabilities. The resulting states of being, of consciousness, teach one the basic truth about one's own equipment as follows:

> In the province of the mind, what one believes to be true is true or becomes true, within certain limits to be found experientially and experimentally. These limits are further beliefs to be transcended. In the mind, there are no limits. (Lilly, 1972).

In the province of the mind is the region of one's models, of the alone self, of memory, of the metaprograms. What of the region which includes one's body, other's bodies? Here there are definite limits.

In the network of bodies, one's own connected with others for bodily survival-procreation-creation, there is another kind of information:

> In the province of connected minds, what the network believes to be true, either is true or becomes true within certain limits to be found experientially and experimentally. These limits are further beliefs to be transcended. In the network's mind there are no limits.

But, once again, the bodies of the network housing the minds, the ground on which they rest, the planet's surface, impose definite limits. These limits are to be found experientially and experimentally, agreed upon by special minds, and communicated to the network. The results are called concensus science.

Thus, so far, we have information without limits in one's mind and with agreed-upon limits (possibly unnecessary) in a network of minds. We also have information within definite limits (to be found) with one body and in a network of bodies on a planet.

With this formulation, our scientific problem can be stated very succinctly as follows:

Given a single body and a single mind physically isolated and confined in a completely physically-controlled environment in true solitude, by our present sciences can we satisfactorily account for all inputs and all outputs to and from this mind — biocomputer (i.e., can we truly isolate and confine it?)? Given the properties of the software-mind of this biocomputer outlined above, is it probable that we can find, discover, or invent inputs-outputs not yet in our concensus science? Does this center of consciousness receive-transmit information by at present unknown modes of communication? Does this center of consciousness stay in the isolated confined biocomputer?

In this book I try to show you where I am in this search and research. In previous books I have dealt with personal experiences. Here I deal with theory and methods, metaprograms and programs.

J.C.L.

February 1972
Los Angeles, California

¤ Preface to First Edition

This work is the result of several years of personal effort to try to understand the various paradoxes of the mind and the brain and their relationships. It is felt that the basic premises presented in this work may help resolve some of the philosophical and theoretical difficulties which arise when one uses other viewpoints and other basic beliefs.

Some of the major philosophical puzzles are concerned with existence of self, with the relation of the self to the brain, the self to the mind, and self to other minds, the existence or non-existence of an immortal part of the self, and the creation of and the belief in various powerful phantasies in these areas of thought.

In Man there is a basic need for imagining wish-fulfillments. Man's wishful thinking becomes interwoven among his best science and even his best philosophy. For the intellectual and the emotional advancement of each of us we need certain kinds of ideals. We also need ways of thinking which look as straight at the *inner* realities as at the physical-chemical-biological *outer* realities. We need truly objective philosophical analysis inside ourselves as well as outside ourselves. This work is a summary of a current position in progress to try to attain objectivity and impartiality with respect to the innermost realities.

One might well ask where is such theory applicable? Once mastered, it may be directly applied in self-analysis. If one remembers that one's self is a feedback-cause with other human beings, one can start at this personal end of the system and achieve beginnings of *interhuman* analysis by analyzing one's self first. If successful, one may see one's self operating in improved fashions with other people, as judged by one's self and, much later, as judged by others. The reflections of one's intellectual and emotional growth later may begin to be distributed and are then seen operating in one's interhuman transactions — with one's wife, children, relatives, colleagues, and professional and business contacts.

The persons who can understand and absorb this kind of theory need understand over a broad intellectual and emotional front. Each one needs understanding and training in depth in multiple fields of human endeavor. Those persons who probably can understand it best are the *general scientists.* * Among those in this group to whom I have presented the theory, there was immediate understanding and an immediate grasping of the basic fundamentals and of the consequence of the theory.

A second group who have no difficulty with the *computer* aspects but who may have difficulty with the *subjective* aspects is that large group of young people who are becoming immersed more and more in computers, their use and programing. A few of these may have the necessary biological and psychoanalytic background to understand this viewpoint. Additional training may be given to these few in self-analysis itself.

Several members of a third group may find it useful with further study, the classically trained psychoanalytic scientists.

---

* A general scientist (as defined for purposes of this discussion) is a person trained in the scientific method and trained in watching his own mind operate and correcting his scientific as well as philosophical and pragmatic errors. In a sense he is a scientist who is willing to study more than just one narrow speciality in an attempt to grasp as much knowledge as he can under the circumstances from other fields than his own. He has a grasp of symbolic logic and of mathematics which he can apply to problems other than his own scientific speciality.

The psychoanalytic group may have difficulties in that very few are trained in the *general purpose* types of thinking involved in *general purpose* computers.

There are difficulties in the way of a multidisciplinary group, as a group, to use this theory. It seems necessary that each individual absorb the necessary kinds of thinking and kinds of motivations involved in each of the fields represented. Members of such groups can motivate one another to do individual learning in these areas and can help one another learn in these various areas. It is up to each responsible individual to absorb enough to gain understanding on the levels presented.

As with most insights into the *innermost realities*, it is felt that many of the advantages of this viewpoint cannot be seen directly until this way of thinking is absorbed into one's mind. The thinking machinery itself is at stake here. Once absorbed and understood I have found it possible to see that the properties and the operations of one's mind in many different states can be accounted for somewhat more satisfactorily. With the resulting increased control over conscious thinking and preconscious computations, with the newly enhanced respect for one's fixed unconscious (as if built-in) programs, the integration of one's self with the deeper inner realities becomes more satisfactory.

The theory is phrased in definite statements. However, it is not intended that the reader take this version as definitive, final, completed, or closed. Each of these definite statements is to be accepted only as a working hypothesis as currently presented by the author. My aim is not to make a new final philosophy, a new religion, or a new rigid way of approaching man's intellectual life. My aim is to increase the flexibility, the power, and the objectivity of our currently limited mind and its knowledge of itself. We have come a long way from the lowly primate to our present level. (However, we have a long way to go to realize the best obtainable from ourselves.) One has only to look at the inadequacies of Man's treatment of Man, and see how far we must go if we are to survive as a progressing species with better control of our battling animalistic superstitious levels.

It is expected that this theory will be useful in understanding and in programming not only one's self but other minds as well. Enhancement of the very human depths of communication with other minds may be approached. The current limits and the attainable limits for education, for reprogramming, for therapy and for cooperative efforts of all sorts between men, may be aided in the terms here presented. This is at least a hope of the author. Only time and use of this kind of thinking can test out the further working hypothesis.

One fact which must be appreciated for applying this theory is the essential individual uniqueness of each of our minds, of each of our brains. It is no easy work to analyze either one's self or someone else. This theory is not, cannot be, a miracle key to a given human mind. It is devilishly hard work digging up enough of the basic facts and enough of the basic programs and metaprograms controlling each mind from within to change its poor operations into better ones. This theory can help one to sort out and arrange stored information and facts into more effective patterns for change. But the basic investigation of self or of other selves is not easy or fast. Our built-in prejudices, biases, repressions and denials fight against understanding. Our Unconscious automatically controls our behavior. Eventually we may be able to progress farther. It may take several generations of those willing to work on these problems.

I have a question about the wisdom of publishing too much of me, myself. I hesitate to publish in this small work certain personal observations in depth and in detail. If the society in which we live were more ideal, I might so publish. (Possibly in such an ideal society there might be no need for such work.) I do not know the answer, nor will I espouse the cause of those who feel they do know either the yes or the no answer. Frankly, I am an explorer in this area. My ambition is to be free to **explore**, not to **exploit**. I share what I experience because that is my profession — to search, to find, to discuss, and to write within Science what I find. Let others use what I may be privileged to find in their own professions, businesses, and/or pursuits. I have found that as soon as I *go commercial, go political*, or any other motivational endeavor, I lose what I personally prize most — my objectivity, my dispassionate appraisal, my freedom to explore the mind within my own particular limits. To make money, to cure someone, to rule, to be elected, to grant money, to be a specialist in one science are all necessary and grand human enterprises needing persons of high intellectual and dedicated maturity. I do not seem to be of those (maybe I do or did not choose to be). In the United States of America in 1966, to insist on the explorer's role in the region of Man's innermost mind is to insist on being intellectually unconventional and to espouse a region of endeavor of research difficult to support. Grants for scientific research tend to be awarded by specialists to specialists; this is true in medical sciences as well as others. This current work cuts through too many specialties for that kind of support. I hope someday that approaches such as this one can be supported on their own merit.

Respect for the Unknown is hard to come by. Support for a science devoted to the Innermost Unknowns is needed.

METATHEORETICAL CONSIDERATIONS

In general there are two opposing and different schools of thought on the basic origins of systems of thought or systems of mathematics. In a simplified way these two extreme positions can be summarized as follows:

1. In the first position one makes the metatheoretical assumption that a given system of thinking is based upon irre-

ducible postulates — the basic beliefs of the systems. All consequences and all manipulations of the thinking machine are then merely elaborations of, combinations of, these assumptions operating upon data derived from the mind and/or from the external world. This is called the *formalistic* school. This school assumes that one can, with sufficiently sophisticated methods, find those postulates which are motivating and directing a given mind in its operations. A further metatheoretical assumption is that once one finds this set of postulates that then one can account for all of the operations of that mind. (Whitehead and Russell, 1927; Carnap, 1942-46; Tarski, 1946.)

2. The opposing school at the opposite end of a spectrum of schools, as it were, makes the metatheoretical assumption that thinking systems arise from intuitive, essentially unknowable, substrates of mental operations (Hilbert, 1950). This school states that new kinds of thinking are created from unknown sources. Further, one is not able to arrive at all of the basic assumptions on which systems of thinking operate. Many of the assumptions from this point of view must be forever hidden from the thinker. Thus in this view the origins of thinking are wide open. With this metatheoretical assumption one can then conceive of the existence in the future of presently inconceivable systems of thought.

3. There is an intermediate position between these two extremes in which one assumes the existence of both kinds and that each of these two extremes has something to offer. Thus one can select kinds of thinking which are subject to formalistic analysis and formalistic synthesis based upon basic beliefs. But this does not include all thinking. Some kinds continue to be based in unknown areas, sources, and methods. Metatheoretical selection is

being done by selection of the formal kind of thinking from a large universe of other possibilities. This position does not state that the origins of the basic beliefs are completely specifiable. However, once some related basic beliefs are found to exist, a limited system of rules of combination of the basic beliefs giving internally consistent logical results can be devised for limited use of that system. This organization into a limited integral system of thinking and the selection of those basic beliefs which naturally fit into such systems of thinking, is a way of dividing off this territory.

Among many other metatheoretical ways of looking at one's own thinking machine and its activities is one which considers the unknown origins of basic beliefs and finding those whose origins are unknown. The whole problem of origin and the whole problem of how one constructs basic beliefs is at stake here.

If one takes a naturally occurring, thinking mind and obtains a sufficiently large sample of its thinking, one can have a metatheoretical faith that one can then find the basic beliefs and their origins. I am not too sure that such metatheoretical faith in one's ability to adequately observe, adequately record, and adequately analyze mental events and construct them into logical explanations is warranted. With certain areas of thinking one can do this, with certain kinds of minds one can do this, but are not these the minds which have been organized along the known metatheoretical pathways? Are not these the minds which believe implicitly in metatheoretical terms in a basic set of beliefs and operate with them in an obvious direct logical fashion?

May it not be better to conceive of minds and of criteria of excellence for *general purpose minds* in which one plugs in, as it were, metatheoretical positions which do not have only this area of applied formalism. In certain areas of thinking, of course, it is necessary to have a set of basic beliefs including those of the rules of various kinds of *games* that one must play in the external physical reality and in the social reality.* One can play these at different levels of abstraction with more or less excellence at playing, with or without dedication, etc. Interlock with external reality has its own requirements, not just those of the mind itself. In this paper external reality is not the area of major emphasis as can be seen in other portions of the paper. The interest of the author is more in the thinking machine itself, unencumbered. During those times when it is unencumbered by the necessities of interlock with other computers and/or with an external reality, its noninterlock structure can be studied. A given mind seen in pure culture by itself in profound physical isolation and in solitude is the raw material for our investigation (Lilly, 1956).

Thus our major interests are in those metatheoretical positions which remain as open as possible to reasonable explanation and reasonable models of the thinking processes of the origins of beliefs, of the origins of self, the organization of self with respect to the rest of the mind, and the kinds of permissible transformations of self which are reversible, flexible, and introduce new and more effective ways of thinking.

Is one of the sum and substance of one's experience, of one's genetics, genic inheritance, of one's modeling of other humans and of other animals and of plants, or is one something in addition to this? As we chip away at this major question of existence of self, as men have chipped away at this question over the millenia, we find that this kind of question and the attempt to answer it have led to new understandings, new mathematics, new sciences, new points of view and new human activities. If one attempts to conceive of one's self as having gone through another kind of evolution other than that of the

---

*Von Neumann & Morgenstern.

human, if one attempts to conceive of himself having lived in an environment different from the social one that we have been exposed to, or if one attempts to imagine having evolved as an organism with the same (or greater) degree of intelligence in the sea or on a planet nearer the sun or farther from the sun, one realizes the essentially *prejudiced* nature of one's self. Let one carefully consider, for example, the genic mutations leading to different human form, structure, function and mental set. One metatheoretical position is that all such mutations in their proper combination exposed to the proper environment (of which there must be millions of possibilities) can survive and progress. In other words, even those mutations which are lethal now, may have survival value under special new and different conditions.

If there is any truth in this statement then we should be doing a whole set of experiments on the adaptability and the seeking of the proper environment, proper peculiar diets, proper relation of sleep-wakefulness, light to dark, amount of various kinds of radiation, amount of noise, amount of motion, and so forth for mutants at each stage in their life cycle. In other words, we should experiment with all of the vast parameters in which we have evolved and their variations in order to seek optimal survival values of these for the embryo, fetuses and children who do not survive under our peculiarly narrow range of values of these parameters. To change *lethals* to *optimals* seems possible and even probable with imaginative and thorough research.

Our genetic code with all its possible variations is a *general purpose construction kit* for a vast set of organisms, only a few examples of which we see in the adult human population in all races around the world. This molecular construction kit for organisms (through the exigencies of matings, of early embryonic development and growth, of the conditions imposed by mother, her diet and physical and social surroundings) gives rise to organisms which test experimentally the conditions imposed upon them and test how well the particular combination and particular values in their genic code are combined to form an integral complete organism for coping with that particular environment and those particular organisms found in that environment (including bacteria and viruses).

One can conceive of an infinity of other environments populated with other viruses, bacteria, and complex organisms in which Man as such could not survive in his present form. One could also conceive of our genetic code (as given) generating organisms who could and would survive and progress under those new conditions.

Until we have thoroughly explored this genetic code, until we can specify the organism and the conditions under which it can reach maturity, and become an integral individual, we will not have the data necessary for specifying all of the characteristics of the human computer which are brought to the adult from the sperm-egg combination.

We have not tested our own range of adaptability (as integral adults) to all possible environments. Scientifically we have little experience with the extreme; we know something of the extremes of temperature, of air and of water in which we can survive. We know something of the radiation limits within which we can survive. We know something of the oxygen concentrations in the air that we breathe, we know something of the light levels within which we can function. We know a little of the sound levels in which we can function, and so forth. We are beginning to see how the environment interlocks with our computer and changes its functioning. We are beginning to see how certain kinds of experiences with these conditions set up rules which we call *physical science* within our own minds. We are beginning to see how, if we change the external conditions, in a limited way within a limited piece of apparatus, that these rules must be changed in order to understand how we can model these changed conditions and the way that atoms, molecules, radiation and space behave, in our own minds. This century has seen vast advances in our modeling of radiation, material particles of matter, space, stars, galaxies, solid materials, liquids, and our small modifications of all of these. This century, however, has not seen a similar gain in our understanding of the operations of our own minds, of the essential origins of thinking, and of those conditions under which we can elect to create new thinking machines within our minds.

In this century we have begun to appreciate some of the powerful and special organizations of matter which are our essential organisms. The advances in the last fifty years in biochemistry, in genetics, and in biophysics and molecular biology are the beginnings of a new control of these distributions of matter within ourselves.

Schrödinger* said that the chromosome (which contains the linear genetic code) to a physicist is a linear two-dimensional solid; along its length it has a great strength and yet it is a flexible chain which can move and which can be split down the middle during mitosis. These carriers of the orders for our ultimate structure as an integral adult, their essential immortality in being passed from one individual to the next in creating the next individual in line, should not be neglected in any theory of the operation of our mind. It may be that our basic beliefs, the unique ones of each one of us, can be found by careful correlations between our essentially unique genic maps and our thinking limits. It may be that the kinds and levels of thinking of which each of us is capable is essentially determined by the genes which are contained in each of us. It may be that each of our private languages is genically determined. Even if this is true, that there is genic determinism in regard to our thinking machines, we are not yet at the point at which we can specify the levels of abstraction and the cognitional and theoretical entities which are genically controlled.

---

*Schrödinger (1945).

If we can free ourselves from the effects on our thinking machine of storage of material from the external world, if we can free ourselves up from the effects of storage of metaprograms which direct our thinking, programs devised by others and fed to us during our learning years, we may be able to see the outline and the essential variables which are genically determined. This is an immensely difficult area for research. It will require the services of many talented individuals considering their own thinking processes, combined with a detailed knowledge of their genic structure and their genic predecessors.

Of course in this discussion we are entering into difficulties brought about by the phenotype-genotype differences. These will have to be taken into account as will all of the other mechanisms so laboriously worked out and discovered in the science of genetics. But these rules of genetics must not be limiting in the metatheory; they must enter as part of the knowledge of these talented individuals and at the correct level of abstraction for seeking the patterns of thinking which are genically controlled.

This *genic determinism of thinking* can turn out to be a will-o-the-wisp. It may be that in the subsequent development of the computer it has become so general purpose that the original genetic factors and the genes are no longer of importance. Even as one can construct a very very large computer of solid state parts or of vacuum tube parts or of biological parts, it makes little difference as long as the total size, the excellence of the connections and the kinds of connections are such that one can obtain a general purpose net result from the particular machine. So may we possibly cancel out genic differences. So may each one of us, as it were, attain the same kinds of learning and the same kind of thinking machine little modified by genic differences.

I do not wish to take sides on these issues. I merely wish to say that if one is to take an impartial and dispassionate view, one cannot afford to espouse deeply any fixed pattern of thinking with regard to these matters. I would prefer to see talented individuals with large mental capabilities investigating their own minds to the very depths. I want to aid these individuals in their communication of the results to others, with similar yet different talents. I believe that by using certain methods and means, some of which are presented in this work, that truly talented and dedicated individuals can forge, find, and devise new ways of looking at our minds, which are truly scientific, intellectually economical, and interactively creative. Consider, for example, the case of the fictitious individual created by the group of mathematicians masquerading under the name of *Dr. Nicholas Bourbaki.*

This group of mathematicians in order to create a mathematics or sets of mathematics beyond the capacity of any one individual, held meetings three times a year and exchanged ideas, then went off and worked separately. The resulting papers were published under a pseudonym because the products of this work were felt to be a group result beyond any one individual's contribution.

Whether or not this group was greater than or lesser than a single human mind, operating in isolation on similar materials, will not be known for some time. It may be that the *human computer interlock* achieved among these mathematicians created a new entity greater than any one of them in regard to modes of thinking, complexity of thinking, and creative new ideas. Certain kinds of things that Man does of necessity require tremendous amounts of cooperation among very large numbers of individuals. Such accomplishments are beyond any one individual and are a product only of the group effort. This is true, for example, in building the Empire State Building, a subway system, a railroad system, an airline, a large industrial factory, etc. In each of these cases there is a rearrangement of external realities, a setting up of a communication network between many individuals and a dedication of each of these individuals to the purposes of the organization of which they are a part. This is probably the greatest accomplishment of our industrial, military, educational and religious efforts in this century. Man's effective interlock with other men can accomplish certain kinds of things beyond any individual.

However, in certain areas, gifted, talented, intelligent individuals seem to function almost autonomously as solitudinous computers giving rise to new findings. This is seen in the case of the mathematical geniuses raised in isolation. One is almost afraid to educate such people for fear that they will lose their general purpose nature and their ability to make original creative contributions. Somehow or other they have escaped interlock into Man's ever more pervasive social organizations and their demands. As in the case of the creative physicist Moseley, who was drafted and killed in World War I, such talent can be thrown away by the operations of the necessity of interlock in our society.

There is a point of view in the modern world and there are divisions among intellectuals which are wasting our use of talent and genius. There are antithetical philosophies which cause diversive intellectual activities. It may be that such conflict is necessary for the intellectual advancement of each individual. It may also be completely superfluous and nonsensical. C. P. Snow has pointed out in his writings (especially those about the *two cultures*) that one kind of social dichotomy about which I speak. The value systems of each intellectual reflect his prejudices, his biases, his blindnesses, as well as his areas of competence. It seems to be a very foolish maneuver to take that which one knows, that in which one is excellent and raise it above the general intellectual level of all other intellectuals. One technique of raising what one and one's most intimate colleagues know above the surrounding intellectual terrain is to literally dig an intellectual moat around one's field of activity. To dig this moat one demeans and denigrates areas of knowledge and individuals in those fields surrounding one's own field. This kind of activity seems to be almost built-in in our structure as biological organisms.

J.C.L.
St. Thomas, U.S. Virgin Islands, 1967

◻ Introduction

> "The general (purpose) computer is. . .a machine
> in which the operator can prescribe, for any internal
> state of the machine and for any given condition
> affecting it, what state it shall go to next. . .All
> behaviors are at the operator's disposal. A program
> . . .with the machine forms a mechanism that will
> show (any thinkable) behavior. This generalization
> has largely solved the main problem of the brain
> so far as its objective behavior is concerned; the
> nature of its subjective aspects may be left to the
> next generation, if only to reassure them that there
> are still major scientific worlds left to conquer."
> (W. Ross Ashby, "What Is Mind?" in *Theories of
> the Mind*, Macmillan, New York, 1962.)

The relations of the activities of the brain to the subjective
life in the mind have long been an arguable puzzle. In this
century some advances in the reciprocal fields of study of each
aspect of the question apparently can begin to clear up some of
the dilemmas. This is a report of a theory and its use which is

1

intended to attempt to link operationally, the
   (a) mental subjective aspects,
   (b) neuronal circuit activities,
   (c) biochemistry, and
   (d) observable behavioral variables.
The sources of information used by the author are mainly
   (1) the results and syntheses of his own experiments on the CNS* and the behavior of animals,
   (2) the experiences and results of experiments in profound physical isolation on himself,
   (3) his own psychoanalytic work on himself and others,
   (4) his studies and experience with the design, construction, operation and programming of electronic solid state digital stored-program computers,
   (5) studies of analogue computers for the analysis and conversion of voice frequency spectra for man and for dolphin and the on-line computation of multiple continuous data sources,
   (6) studies and experiments in neuropsychopharmacology,
   (7) research on and with communication with humans, with dolphins, and with both,
   (8) study of certain literature in biology (B), logic (L), neuropsychopharmacology (N), brain and mind models (M), communication (T), psychoanalysis (P), computers (C), psychology (O), psychiatry (I), and hypnosis (H) (see References and Bibliography).

The introduction of open-minded, multiple-level, continuously developing, on-line, operational, dynamic, economical, expanding, structural-functional, field-jumping, field-ignoring theory is needed. The applications of this theory extend from the atomic-molecular-membranes-cell levels, though cell aggregational levels, total behavior and mental-cognitive levels of the single organism of large brain size, and to dyadic and larger groups of such individuals.

---

* Central nervous system

3

BASIC ASSUMPTIONS (Table 2, Figs. 4 & 5)

The basic assumptions are as follows:

1. The human brain is assumed to be an immense biocomputer, several thousands of times larger than any constructed by Man from non-biological components by 1965.

    The numbers of neurons in the human brain are variously estimated at 13 billions (1.3 times ten to the tenth) with approximately five times that many glial cells. This computer operates continuously throughout all of its parts and does literally millions of computations in parallel simultaneously. It has approximately two million visual inputs and one hundred thousand acoustic inputs. It is hard to compare the operations of such a magnificent computer to any artificial ones existing today because of its very advanced and sophisticated construction.

2. Certain properties of this computer are known, others are yet to be found. One of these properties obviously is a very large memory storage. Another is control over hundreds of thousands of outputs in a coordinated and programmed fashion. Other examples are the storage and evocation of all those complex behaviors and perceptions known as speech, hearing and language. Some of the more unusual properties of this computer are given further along in this paper.

3. Certain programs are built-in, within the difficult-to-modify parts of the (macro- and micro-) structure of the brain itself. At the lowest possible level such programs which are built-in are those of feeding, eating, sex, avoidance and approach programs, certain kinds of fears, pains, etc.

4. Programs vary in their permanence, some are apparently evanescent and erasable, others operate without apparent

change for tens of years. Among the evanescent and erasable programs one might categorize the ability to use visual projection in the service of one's own thinking. One finds this ability with a very high incidence among children and a very low incidence among adults. An example of a program operating without change for tens of years one can show handwriting, over a long series of years, to maintain its own unique patterns.

5. Programs are acquirable throughout life. Apparently no matter how old a person is, there is still a possibility of acquiring new habits. The difficulties of acquisition may increase with age, however, it is not too sure that this is correct. The problem may not be with acquiring programs so much as a decrease in the motivation for acquiring programs.

6. The young newly growing computer acquires programs as its structure expands: some of these take on the appearance of built-in permanence. An example of such acquisition of programs in a child is in the pronunciation of words. Once it agrees with those of the parents the pronunciation is very difficult to change later, i.e., there is really no great motivation for the child to change a particular pronunciation when it is satisfactory to those who listen.

7. Some of the programs of the young growing computer are in the inherited genetic code; how these become active and to what extent is known only in a few biochemical-behavioral cases, at variance with the expectable and usual patterns of development. The so-called Mongoloid phenomenon is inherited and develops at definite times in the individual's life. There are several other interesting clinical entities which appear to be genetically determined. To elicit the full potential of the young growing computer

requires special environments to avoid negative anti-growth kinds of programs being inserted in the young computer early.

8. The inherited genetic programs place the upper and the lower bounds on the total real performance and on the potential performance of the computer at each instant of its life span. Once again we are assuming that the best environment is presented to the young organism at each part of its life span. It is not meant to imply that such an environment currently is being achieved. This basic assumption seems highly probable but would be very difficult to test.

9. The major problems of the research which are of interest to the author center on the erasability, modifiability, and creatability of programs. In other words, I am interested in the processes of finding metaprograms (and methods and substances) which control, change, and create the basic metaprograms of the human computer. It is not known whether one can really erase any program. Conflicting schools of thought go from the extremes that *one stores everything within the computer and never erases it* to *only the important aspects and functions are stored in the computer* and hence, there is no problem of erasing. Modifications of already existing programs can be done with more or less success. The creation of new programs is a difficult assignment. How can one recognize a new program once it is created? This new program may merely be a variation on already stored programs.

10. To date some of the metaprograms are unsatisfactory (educational methods for the very young, for example). It is doubtful if any metaprogram is fully satisfactory to the inquiring mind. Some are assumed to be provisionally

satisfactory for current heuristic reasons. To keep an open mind and at the same time a firm enough belief in certain essential metaprograms is not easy; in a sense we are all victims of the previous metaprograms which have been laid down by other humans long before us.

11. The human computer has *general purpose* properties within its limits. The definition of *general purpose* implies the ability to attack problems that differ not only in quantitative degree of complexity but also that differ qualitatively in the levels of abstraction in the content dealt with. One can shift rapidly one's mind and its attention from one area of human activity to another with very little delay in the reprogramming of one's self to the new activity. The broader the front of such reprogramming the more general purpose the computer is. The ability to move from the interhuman business world to the laboratory world of the scientist would be an example of a fairly general purpose computer.

12. **The human computer has *stored program* properties.** A stored program is a set of instructions which are placed in the memory storage system of the computer and which control the computer when orders are given for that program to be activated. The activator can either be another system within the same computer, or someone, or some situation outside the computer.

13. **The human computer, within limits yet to be defined, has "self-programming" properties, and *other persons-programming* properties.** This assumption follows naturally from the previous one but brings in the systems within the mind which operate at one level of abstraction above that of programming. As is shown in Fig. 1, one literally has to talk about self-metaprogramming as well as self-programming. This does not imply that the whole computer can be

thought of as **the self**. Only small portions of the systems operating at a given instant are taken up by the self-meta-programs. In other words there has to be room for the huge store of programs themselves, of already built-in circuitry for instinctual processes, etc. All of these exist in addition to others leaving only a portion of the circuitry available for the self-metaprograms. The next section emphasizes this aspect.

14. This computer has *self-metaprogramming* properties, with limits determinable and to be determined. (Note: **self-meta-programming is done consciously in metacommand language. The resulting programming then starts and continues below the threshold of awareness.**) Similarly, each computer has a certain level of ability in **metaprogramming others-not-self**.

15. The older classifications of fields of human endeavor and of science are redefinable with this view of the human brain and the human mind. For example, the term *suggestibility* has often been used in a limited context of programming and of being programmed by someone outside. Hypnotic phenomena are seen when a given computer allows itself to be more or less completely programmed by another one. *Metaprogramming* is considered a more inclusive term than *suggestibility*. Metaprogramming considers sources, inputs, outputs, and central processes rather than just the end result of the process (see Fig. 1). Suggestibility names only the property of receiving orders and carrying them out rather than considering the sources, inputs, outputs, and central processes (ref. H. Bernheim, Clark Hull).

16. The mind is defined as the sum total of all the programs and the metaprograms of a given human computer, whether or not they are immediately elicitable, detectable, and

visibly operational to the self or to others. (Thus, in alternative terminology, the mind includes unconscious and instinctual programs.) This definition and basic assumption has various heuristic advantages over the older terminologies and concepts. The mind-brain dichotomy is no longer necessary with this new set of definitions. **The mind is the sum of the programs and metaprograms, i.e., the software of the human computer**.

17. The brain is defined as the visible palpable living set of structures to be included in the human computer; the computer's real boundaries in the body are yet to be fully described (biochemical and endocrinological feedback from target organs, for example). The boundary of the brain, of course, may be considered as the limits of the extensions of the central nervous system into the periphery. One would include here also the so-called *autonomic* nervous system as well as the CNS.

18. There is in certain fields of human thinking and endeavor, a necessity to have a third entity, sometimes including, sometimes not needing the brain-mind-computer; commonly this entity is defined as existing by theologians and other persons interested in religion. Whether the term "spirit" or "soul" or other is used is immaterial in this framework. Such terms inevitably come up in the discussion of the ultimate meanings of existence, the origins of the brain-mind computers, the termination or the destinations of self after bodily death, and the existence or non-existence of minds greater than ours, within or outside of brain-computers. This extra-brain-mind-computer entity can be included in this theory if and when needed. (I agree that such assumptions may be needed to give overall meaning to the whole of Man. Religion is an area for experimental

science. Work starts in this area with the basic assumptions of William James, the great psychologist. The definitions in this area of this theory may be expanded in the future. Some compound term like "brain-mind-spirit-computer may be developed at that time.) There is still the problem of the existence theorem to be satisfied in regard to this third entity. There are some persons who assume it exists; there are others who assume it does not exist.

19. **Certain chemical substances have programmatic and/or metaprogrammatic effects, i.e., they change the operations of the computer, some at the programmatic level and some at the metaprogrammatic level.** Some substances which are of interest at the metaprogrammatic level are those that allow reprogramming, and those that allow and facilitate modifications of the metaprograms. (The old terms for these substances are loaded with diagnostic, therapeutic, medical, moral, ethical, and legal connotations.) To be scientifically useful the social connotations are removed. Such terms as "psychopharmacologically active drugs," "psychotomimetics," "tranquilizers," "narcotics," "drugs," "anaesthetics," "analgesics," etc. are used in a new theory without the therapeutic, diagnostic, moral, ethical, and legal connotations; all of this area should be subjected to careful reevaluation with the new view in mind. Applications of good theory to the social levels may help to unravel this area of controversy.

For example, the term "reprogramming substances" may be appropriate for compounds like lysergic acid diethylamide. For substances like ethyl alcohol the term "metaprogram-attenuating substances" may be useful. Similarly the theory proposed may be useful in other areas in the classical fields of psychopharmacology, neurophysiology, biochemistry, and psychology, among others. Some of the detailed operations of the brain itself can be operationally organized to show how programs are carried out by excitation-inhibition-disinhibition patterns among and in neural masses and sheets (for example, the reticular activating-inhibiting system, the reward-punishment systems, the cerebral-cortical conditionable systems, etc.). (Tables 3-10, Figs. 8 and 9)

20. It is not intended that I be dogmatic in the new definitions of this version of the theory.

Speed in the recording of the ideas is preferred to perfection of the concepts and deriving the ultimate in internal consistency. As the theory grows, so may grow its accuracy and applicability. It is intended that the theory remains as open-minded as possible without sacrificing specificity in hazy generality. The language chosen is as close to basic English as possible.

As the theory develops, a proper kind of symbolism may be developed to succinctly summarize the points and allow manipulations of the logic to elucidate elaborations of the argument in various cases.

It is known that the common "machine-language" of mammalian brains is not yet discovered. **The self-meta-program language is some individual variation of the basic native language in each specific human case. All of the levels and each level expressed in the self-metaprogram language for self-programming cover very large segments of the total operation of the computer, rather than details of its local operations.** Certain concepts of the operation of computers, once effectively introduced into a given mind-brain-computer, change its metaprograms rapidly. Language now takes on a new precision and power in the programming process.

21. Certain kinds of subjective experience reveal some aspects

of the operations of the computer to the self. Changes in the states of consciousness are helpful in delineating certain aspects of the bounds and the limits of these operations. Inspection of areas of stored data and programs not normally available is made possible by special techniques. **Special aspects and areas of stored programs can be visualized, felt, heard, lived through or replayed, or otherwise elicited from memory storage by means of special techniques and special instructions.** The evocation can be confined to one or any number of sensory modes, with or without motor replay simultaneously.

22. After and even during evocation from storage, within certain limits, desired attenuations, corrections, additions, and new creations with certain half-lives can be made. These can be done with (fixed but as yet not determinable) half-lives in conscious awareness, and can subsequently be weakened or modified or replaced, to a certain extent to be determined individually. **An unmodifiable half-life can turn up for certain kinds of programs subjected to antithetical metaprograms, i.e., orders to weaken, modify or replace a program act as antithetical metaprograms to already existing programs or metaprograms.**

23. New areas of conscious awareness can be developed, beyond the current conscious comprehension of the self. With courage, fortitude, and perseverance the previously experienced boundaries can be crossed into new territories of subjective awareness and experience. New knowledge, new problems, new puzzles are found in the innermost explorations. Some of these areas may seem to transcend the operations of the mind-brain-computer itself. In these areas there may be a need for the meta-computer mappings; but first the evasions constructed by the computer itself must be found, recognized, and re-programmed. *New* **knowledge**

often turns out to be merely *old and hidden* knowledge after mature contemplative analysis.

24. Some kinds of material evoked from storage seem to have the property of passing back in time beyond the beginning of this brain to previous brains at their same stage of development; there seems to be a passing of specific information from past organisms through the genetic code to the present organism; but, again, this idea may be a convenient evasion, avoiding deeper analysis of self. One cannot make this assumption that storage in memory goes back beyond the sperm-egg combination or even to the sperm-egg combination until a wishful phantasy constructed to avoid analyzing one's self ruthlessly and objectively is eliminated.

25. **Apparently not all programs are revisable.** The reasons seem various; some are held by feedback established with other mind-brain-computers in the life-involvement necessary for procreation, financial survival, and practice of business or profession. Other non-revisable programs are those written in emergencies in the early growth years of the computer. The programs dealing with survivals of the young self sometimes seem to have been written in a hurry in desparate attempts to survive; these seem most intransigent.

26. **Priority lists of programs can function as metaprograms.** Certain programs have more value than others. By making such lists the individual can find desired revision points for rewriting important metaprograms. In other words it is important to determine what is important in one's own life.

27. The basic bodily and mental function programs and their various forms dealt with in verbal-vocal modes (words, speech, etc.) have been described in great detail in the psychoanalytic literature. Evasion, denial, and repression

are varieties of metaprograms dealing with the priority list of programs. **Metaprograms to hide (repress) certain kinds of storage material are commonly found in certain persons.** Such analyses are confined to the verbal-vocal-acoustic modes. **Encounters with other persons in the real world are much more powerful in terms of modifications of programs than either psychoanalysis or self-analysis.** For example learning through sexual intercourse cannot be given through the verbal-vocal mode.

28. The detailed view of certain kinds of non-speech, non-verbal learning programs, i.e., some of the methods of introducing such programs and parts thereof, are exemplified in the work of I. P. Pavlov and of B. F. Skinner. Some of these results are the teaching and the learning of a simple code or language, a code with non-verbal elements (non-vocalized and non-acoustic) with autonomic components (Gordon Pask, 1966). Other motor outputs than the phonation apparatus are used.

29. **The reward-punishment dichotomy or spectrum is critically important within the human computer's operations.** (Figs. 2, 6-8, 10-12 and Tables 3-7)

    The fact of various CNS circuits existing as reward and as "punishment" systems when stimulated by artificial or by natural inputs must be taken into account (Lilly, J. C., 1957, 1958, 1959). The powerful emotional underpinnings of "movement toward" and "movement away" must be included, as well as the acquisition of code symbols for these processes. Such symbols tend to set up the priority hierarchies of basic operational programs in micro-format (non-verbal) and in macro-format (verbal). Too often, "accidental" juxtaposition seems to key off improper hierarchical relations at the outset, with resulting priorities set by "first occurrence" spontaneous configurations, unplanned and unprepared. With a new view and a new approach, with planned "spontaneities" graded by order of occurrence, proper program priorities could be set at the beginning of the computer's life history. **The maintenance of general purpose properties from the early human years to adulthood is a worthwhile metaprogram.**

The positive (pleasure producing) and negative (pain or fear producing) aspects of the programs and metaprograms strike at the very roots of motivational energies for the computer. One aspect of lysergic acid diethylamide is that it can give an overall positive motivational aspect to the individual in the LSD-25 state. This may facilitate program modifications, but it also can facilitate seeking pleasure as a goal of itself.

30. Various special uses of the human computer entail **a principle of the competing use of the limited amount of total available apparatus.** To hold and to display the accepted view of reality in all its detail and at the same time to program another state of consciousness is difficult; there just isn't enough human brain circuitry to do both jobs in detail perfectly. Therefore special conditions give the best use of the whole computer for exploring, displaying, and fully experiencing new states of consciousness; physical isolation (only with special limited stimulation patterns, if any) (Lilly, 1956) gives the fullest and most complete experiences of the internal explorations. One such extreme condition is profound physical isolation (isothermicity, zero-level visible quanta, sonic levels below threshold, minimum gravitational-resisting unit area forces, minimum internal stimulation intensity, minimum respiration stimulus level, etc.). This condition can give some additional new states of consciousness the "necessary low-level evenness of context" in which to develop. These results are facilitated

by minimizing the necessities for computing the present demands of the physical reality and its calculable present consequences *(physical reality programs).*

Using this principle of the competitive use of portions of the available brain it is important to understand why, for example, a large amount of *hallucinating* would not be permissible in our present society. If a person is actively projecting visual images in three dimensions from his stored programs, he may not have enough of his brain functioning in ordinary modes to take care of him with regard to say, gravity, automobiles, and similar hazards. He may become so involved in the projection in the visual field that the inputs from reality itself have to be sacrificed and their quality reduced. It is apparently this danger which teaches us to inhibit *hallucinations* (i.e., visual projection displays) in the very young children.

31. The principle of the competitive use of available computer structure has a corollary: **the larger the computer is, the larger the total number of metaprograms and of programs storable, and the larger the space which can be used for one or more of the currently active programs simultaneously operating.** The larger the number of actuable elements in the brain the greater the abilities to simultaneously deal with the current reality program and to reinvoke a past stored-reality program. The quality of the details of the reinvoked program and the quality of the operations in the current physical reality are a direct function of the computer's absolute functional size, all other values being equal.

There may be brains which are large enough to simultaneously project from storage into the visual field and also to function adequately in the outside environment. At least conceptually this is a possibility. This partition of the programs among various modes of operation of course are included in our definition of the general purpose nature of this particular computer.

32. **The "consciousness program" itself is expandable and contractable within the computer's structure within certain limits.** In coma, this program is very nearly inoperative; in ordinary states of awareness it needs a fair fraction of the machinery to function. In expanded states of consciousness the fraction of the total computer devoted to its operation expands to a large value. If the consciousness is sensorially expanded maximally, there is little structure left for motoric initiation of complex interaction and vice versa. If motor initiation is expanded, the sensorial creations are reduced in scope. If neither sensorial nor motor activities are expanded, more room is available for cognition and/or feeling, etc.

33. The steady state values of the fractions of the total computer each devoted to a separate program at a given instant add up to the total value of one. The value of a given fraction can fluctuate with time. The places used in the computer also change.

34. **In general there are delineable major systems of metaprograms and of programs competing for the available circuitry.** The methods of categorizing these competing programs depend on the observer's metaprograms. One system divides the competitors into visual, acoustic, proprioceptive, emotive, inhibitory, excitory, disinhibitory, motor, reflexive, learned, appetitive, pleasurable, and painful. This system is used in neurophysiology and comparative physiology.

35. Another system of classification divides the competing metaprograms and programs into oral, anal, genital, defensive, sublimated, conscious, unconscious, libidinal, aggress-

ive, repressive, substitutive, resistive, tactical, strategic, successful, unsuccessful, passive, feminine, active, masculine, pleasure, pain, regressive, progressive, fixated, ego, id, super-ego, ego ideal. This is the system of classification employed by psychoanalysis.

36. Another system divides the competitors into animal, humanistic, moral, ethical, financial, social, altruistic, professional, free, wealthy, poor, progressive, conservative, liberal, religious, powerful, weak, political, medical, legal, economical, national, local, engineering, scientific, mathematical, educational, humanistic, childlike, adolescent, mature, wise, foolish, superficial, deep, profound, thorough, etc. This is a classification which is employed in general by humanitarians and intellectuals.

37. The classifications of metaprograms and/or of programs by the above methods illustrate some useful principles to be included. There is probably a set of better schemes than any of the above ones. Such new systematizations are needed; the principles in this theory may be useful in setting them up at each and every level of functioning of the computer.

Use of Projection-Display Techniques
in Deep Self-Analysis with
Lysergic Acid Diethylamide (LSD-25)

The use of the psychedelic agents (such as LSD-25) in the human subject shows certain properties of these substances in changing the computer's operations in certain ways. Some of these changes are mentioned above in passing; a summary of those found in the LSD state empirically are as follows:

1. **The self-metaprogram can make instructions to create special states of the computer;** many of these special states have been described in the literature on hypnosis.

2. These instructions are carried out with relatively short delays (minutes). The delays of course will vary with the complexity of the task which is being programmed into the computer. It also is a previous history of this same kind of programming: the more often it has been done the easier it is to do again and the less time it takes.

3. **Only *taboo* or *forbidden* programs are not fully constructed:** there are peculiar gaps which give away the fact that there are forbidden areas. Within realizable limits most other programs can be produced.

4. When one first does enter into the storage systems the way the material is held in the dynamic storage is entirely strange to one's conscious self.

5. Production of *displays* of data patterns, of instructions, or storage contents, or of current problems can be realized through such instructions. [A "display" is any visual (or acoustic, or tactile, etc.) plotting of a set of discriminative variables in any number of dimensions of the currently available materials.] The motivational sign and intensity can be varied in any of these displays under special orders.

6. More or less complete re-plays of past experiences important in current computations can be programmed from storage; the calendar objective time of original occurrence seems a not too important aspect of the filing system; the level of maturation of the computer at the time of original occurrence is of greater import.

7. Stored or filed occurrences, filed instructions, filed programs vary in the amount and specificity of positive and/or negative affect-feeling-emotion attached to each. If too negative (evil, harmful, fearful) an emotional charge is attached, re-play can allow readjustment toward the positive end of the motivation-feeling-emotion spectrum. With the LSD-25 state the negative or the positive charge can be changed to neutral or to its opposite by special instructions. However, since most people wish to avoid the negative and encourage the positive once they obtain control over programming they tend to put a positive charge even on programs and metaprograms and the processes of creating them. (A chemical change may take place in signal storage (Fig. 1) as the sign of the motivational process shifts from negative to positive.)

The following description gives examples of the successful uses of and the results with the freedom to program new instructions during the LSD state. It is to be emphasized for those who have not seen the phenomena within themselves that this kind of manipulation and control of one's own programs and its rather dramatic presentation to one's self is apparently not achievable outside of the use of LSD-25. This amount of control can be said to resemble other ways of achieving control and visual projection but in actual intensity I know of no other way to achieve it. Hypnosis is a possible exception.

In some cases during the eight or so possible hours of the special states of consciousness achievable with the help of LSD-25, the use of visually projected images to aid in seeing the nature of one's own defensive, evasive, and idealization mechanisms can be realized. By means of a mirror for the careful inspection of the body in the external reality (the whole body or the face alone) it is possible to induce a special state of consciousness (or a special program or metaprogram in the use of perception circuitry) in which remembered or unconsciously stored images of self or of others appear on or in place of the body image. Such stored images can be selected within certain limits, manipulated within other limits, or allowed to occur in a free-association context, appearing as parallels of the current thought-stream. The orders to self for the appearance of these phenomena may resemble the post-hypnotic suggestion instructions given during auto-hypnosis, the metaprogrammatic instructions to a very large computer for a certain type of display program with special content to be displayed, and the orders to a large organization to produce a play with many actors operating in one place in space, one after the other, each with an assigned role not necessarily specified in detail. For periods of 30 or so minutes of objective time such projections can be maintained and worked with in the self-analysis context; at the end of this time-interval some fatigue is noted with subsequent stopping of the display. Re-evocation can be achieved by a period of rest from this and similar tasks for a period of 15 minutes objective time. Several such periods can be evoked during a single session.

Areas of unconsciously operating taboos, denials and inhibitions are revealed (in negative, as it were) by the absence of appearance of the consciously desired and ordered projections in certain areas. Areas of unconscious elaboration show as projections of great detail and completeness even though no real remembered reality could possibly correspond to the projection. Screen memories (Bertram Lewin, et al.) show in great profusion. As the buried material behind the screen is uncovered, the screen memory disappears.

An apparent defensive maneuver is the *flickering images* phenomena; the new images come at such a rapid rate (2 or 3 per objective second) like a slowed flickering movie that one cannot inspect any one image long enough to recognize its significance. Another alleged evasion is the melting, or mosaic, or distortion maneuver in which images flow in whole or plastically, or are broken up into parts like a mosaic, or parts are interchanged among several stored images at different levels. **The melting, mosaic or distortion of course can be programmed, of itself, under direct orders. It is only considered an evasion when it is not under the control of the self.**

The current affect and its modulation by conscious wishing is immediately shown on the facial expression of the projection despite a lack of change in the objective face itself (proprioceptively, photographically, etc., detected). The projected face and the real face fit together in three dimensions. It is almost as if the perception systems were using the real face and recomputing it to give a different appearance, i.e., if the real face is held neutral then the *projected face* will manipulate the apparent features of the real face with accurate showing of anger, joy, sexual desire, hatred, jealousy, pleasure, pain, fear, psychic mutilation of ego, adoration of self, and several other such emotions. These have been studied by their mirror-projections.

Conflicts can be projected in several ways: the images switch rapidly back and forth between the two conflicting categories, emotions, orders, persons, ideals, or other. Alternatively, parts (disparate parts) of the internalized argument are projected side by side, giving a peculiar stereoscopic depth-in-conflict appearance to the display. Profound fatigue shows by showing *aged* or *diseased* splotchy images.

The negative operations which prevent certain contents reaching access to the display mechanism can be shown to exist by using alternate "acceptable-to-the-ego-ideal" routes to the display program and its projection. For example, material which cannot be projected onto one's own mirrored image, sometimes can be projected onto a color picture of someone else. In some cases the other person in the picture is most suitably and acceptably of the opposite sex (face alone, full body clothed, or unclothed) for the full use of the display of the desired material.

In the proper circumstances a properly selected real person can also serve as the external reality three-dimensional screen onto which material can be projected. This latter "screen" is not a passive one and may say or do something on its own which either changes the projection or invokes a new program (such as the demanding external reality program) which may abolish the whole phenomenon of projection in the visual display itself. When one sees a visual projection onto the face of another person of, say, one's true deeper feelings, the realization may come that this happens to one all the time below the levels of awareness without the special powers attributable to this substance; i.e., there is an already prepared unconscious "display" (which is here allowed access to the visual mechanism by the special conditions) which normally operates in the external reality program with other persons unconsciously or preconsciously. This first-time finding can have therapeutic benefits in the consequent self-analysis of one's human relations.

CORPOREAL FACE

One interesting kind of a projection onto the image of one's own whole body (or onto the real body of another) is the phenomenon of the self-creation of the *corporeal face*. In this phenomenon, one sees a face of a "monstrous being" whose *projected features* are made up on the following real body parts: the real shoulders become the "top of head," mammal areolae become "oculi" (with female, proptosis), navel to "nares," pubes to "mouth," and with male, penis to "lingua." This face, though quite vacuous of itself, can be made quite frightening, sad or happy with proper programming. Once seen, it is easily programmed even with extreme body position changes. Analysis shows, in a particular case, that this face is in storage from very young childhood and was generated/resulted from phantasies about bodies, male and female, threatening/seductive. This projection is useful as a tracer of certain kinds of fears.

THE BLANK SCREEN

The external reality screens for the projection of the display program in the LSD state thus can be arranged in a set with various dimensions relating each to the others. Among these are: the non-self-real persons; motion pictures of these persons in various states; still pictures of the persons; pictures of self from the past, motion and still, three dimensional and flat; the here-and-now three-dimensional color image of one's face and/or body in a mirror; and finally, the eyes-open or eyes-closed blank unlighted or lighted *projection screen*.

The blank projection screen introspectively considered varies depending upon whether the eyes are open or closed. In the dark, in the absolute dark, one can detect differences between the eyes open and the eyes closed blank screen. The eyes open case gives a feeling of depth out beyond the eyes, a feeling of a *real visual space*. In this subject the eyes closed immediately turns the vision to a different *visual space* which seems more internal, more introspective, more subjective. In the LSD-25 state these differences are attenuated in the profound isolation conditions.

The blank screen is the most difficult one to work with but is the least "driving" of the group. **The blank screen interferes least with one's creative efforts**; it takes more program circuitry to create those aspects which can be furnished by the other screens themselves, from the perception mechanisms directly into the projection program itself. The blank screen does not so easily show the "forbidden transitions" except by remaining blank, i.e., more relaxation and freedom to "free associate" with this visual mode is required to project on a blank screen.

At times the cross-model synesthetic projection may help with the blank screen; excitation coming in the objective hearing mechanisms can be converted to excite visual projection. The commonest excitation used here is music; this well-organized patterned input tends to "drive the content by association." For instance, religious music can evoke religious visions constructed in childhood from real pictures, churches and phantasies, etc. Other inputs are voices, one's own real or recorded voice, the voice of another person: these sources can have problems similar to those with the pictures. The high priority program we are calling the *external reality program* may tend to usurp the circuitry and take over from the projection program with pictures or voices of known and valued persons. This effect interrupts the projection and its free association. In the long run the external reality's content and its connections can be shown to be relevant by continued self-analysis, using the usual techniques of psychoanalysis.

Such interruptions depend upon the individual computer and its conflicts in relation to the projection program versus the external reality program. If there is guilt or fear present, the external sources will attract the energy of the computer back to the *external reality*. Alternatively, if the level of excitation from the person in the external reality rises above a certain value, the whole computer will be turned to that particular person and his/her vocal output and his/her behaviors.

Purely random noise may avoid these difficulties; it may be a proper *acoustically lighted blank screen* for cross-model excitation of the visual projections. Initial experiments with in-phase and non-phase noise in the two ears show some new programming possibilities. One pitfall, here, however, is to avoid the initial problem of the programming by the random processes of the noise itself. This tends to result in chaotic programming, i.e., randomness itself can build up to a large intensity within the metaprogramming systems. With adjustment of the acoustic intensity of the two non-phase related noises these effects can be attenuated and the noisily lighted visual screen used for proper projection purposes. Only preliminary experiments have been done in this region as yet.

ZERO LEVEL EXTERNAL REALITY

When sufficient progress with the external reality projection screens of the various kinds (visual, acoustic to visual synesthetic, body image, and others), the elimination or at least maximal attenuation of all modes of stimulation from the external reality allows deeper direct penetration into the unconscious. The rationale here is that **more circuitry in one's huge computer is freed up from the external excitation programs and hence more can be devoted to the internal cognitive reality and its analysis.** The projection "program" is still used, but in a somewhat different way.

In the maximally attenuated environment (92 to 95°F. isothermal skin, saltwater suspension, zero light levels, near-zero sound levels, without clothes, without wall or floor contacts, in solitude in remote isolation, for several hours), the addition of LSD-25 allows one to see that all the previous experiences with "outside screens" are evasions of deeper penetration of self (and hence are *screens* in the sense of "blocking the view behind," as well as "receiving the projected images").

DEFINITION OF EVASION OF
ANALYSIS OF METAPROGRAMS

In using the term *evasion* it is meant to imply a similar concept to *defensive maneuvers* or *defenses* of the psychoanalytic literature. However, in addition to the content of these concepts, **evasion is defined as** *any program or metaprogram entered upon to avoid, to hide, or to distort a deeper program or metaprogram which is too seductive or too threatening or too chaotic for the self-programmer at that particular time.*

At the beginning in the profound isolation situation many people experience a fear which is an almost *disembodied* fear with no referents in the external reality. With experience this fear can be shown to be a fear of one's own inner unknowns. After a thorough exploration of the various evasive metaprograms, it can be shown that the only thing to fear in this area is fear itself, in overwhelming amounts. With sufficient training it can be shown that one can convert the motivational sign of the experienced emotion from negative to positive. As to whether or not one must go through some of the negative emoting in order to experience enough of the punishing aspects to avoid them is a moot point. A great deal of self-discipline is required in this instance to pursue the negatively tinged programs and metaprograms stored in memory. At times one can detect an almost hedonistic withdrawal from further consideration of unpleasant events and memories. These evasions into pleasure are also evasions of further self-analysis. **As one clears up more and more** areas of unpleasant programs and metaprograms, the increasing amounts of pleasurable programming and metaprogramming and their control can become a very seductive evasion of one's ideal of self-analysis.

It is at this point that too frequent exposure to these conditions must be avoided. Long periods of interlock with the external reality must then be done. Sometimes this may necessitate months of outside work to integrate one's findings with the real world as one has chosen to live in it.

The easily evoked pleasure of the LSD-25 state may become for some persons a major goal. To make sure that one does not get seduced by this induced state of pleasure it is wise to avoid further experiments for several weeks or several months, and re-assert the natural accesses to pleasure in one's external reality. The external reality struggle to obtain pleasure from the environment has rules of its own which must be met realistically and with intelligence and balance. Here it is obvious that discipline in the self-metaprogrammer is absolutely essential. Further progress in self-analysis cannot be made without self-discipline.

With this caution let us return to the profound isolation situation. In the zero level external reality situation the use of any external reality screen can be defined as a defensive maneuver to avoid visualizing or experiencing what one fears most in the deeper levels of one's computer, i.e., in the unconscious. The uses of the screens are necessary and useful steps on the way in and are useful steps to return to for confirmation at later times of the findings. An apparently paradoxical situation thus exists in the profound physical isolation situation. One is pursuing self-analysis and accesses to the keys to pleasure within one's self and keys to lessening the pain and fear in one's self. However, once one has unlocked the pleasure and attenuated the pain one must use the resulting released energies and attach them somehow to the external reality programs and the ideals (supra-self-metaprograms) which one has set up. One does not dissipate all of this pleasure in hedonistic and narcissistic gratification. One of the pitfalls of LSD-25 experiences is exactly this: one has the power now to stay in an expanded state of pleasure, as it were, for several hours. This can become quite seductive and one can become quite lazy and return to this state at every opportunity. However this is not self-analysis, this state is the ecstasy, or bliss, or transcendent state sought by the religious proponents of the use of LSD-25 for *religious purposes*.

These findings are very similar if not identical to those found in classical psychoanalysis. Once repressions and denials are released during the analysis, the access of pleasurable activity increases rapidly. The same temptations exist to become a pleasure-seeking organism; however, this tendency too must be analyzed in the classical situation.

When one compares the classical analytical situation to the solitudinous self-analysis situation one must be quite aware of what has been sacrificed in each case. The advantage of the external analyst being present listening to one producing the material is that one avoids some of the pitfalls of solitude in that some of the above evasions can be pointed out rapidly before one became too involved in them. On the other hand the interpretations of the analyst can be a distraction from pursuing in depth certain aspects of one's own self-analysis. Even solitudinous self-analysis using LSD-25 should be referred back to an external analyst at times when large amounts of powerfully acting unconscious programs have been unearthed. Some programs tend to be *acted out* after profound solitude and isolation experiences, as well as they do during classical analysis. This is one of the risks and the gambles of this technique. This is why one is cautioned to use subjects who have become sophisticated with regard to psychoanalysis itself.

During one's classical psychoanalysis one begins to modify one's computer and the self-programmer to include many aspects of the methods of computation that one's analyst uses. One accumulates as it were a metaprogram of self-analysis which incorporates a good deal of what one's analyst has to offer with regard to one's own computer. In classical psychoanalytic terms one tends to *incorporate many aspects of one's analyst*. Once one has a satisfactorily functioning internal analyst, i.e., an analytical metaprogram for the self-metaprogram, one can be launched on one's own and no longer needs the external analyst to the same degree that one did earlier. One's analysis has proceeded from the analyst outside to the analyst inside.

An analogous situation can be seen in the profound isolation and LSD-25 analysis. The foregoing descriptions of the external screens and external projection methods emphasize the relationship between the computer and the external reality. It also emphasized that the computer was using certain parts of itself for transformations and projections of data from memory into systems stimulated by energies coming from the external world. It was pointed out that such projections were easier to do than when these systems were not excited by energies coming from the outside world. The major reason for failure to be able to project on the *blank screens* or to use the apparatus unexcited by energies coming from the outside world is too great fear of what lies underneath below the levels of awareness in the solitudinous situation. Once a large number of these fears have been analyzed and shown to be peculiarly childlike and childish, one can proceed to the next stage of LSD-25 and isolation combined for analysis.

INNER COGNITION SPACE

As one proceeds from outer or external projection analysis to internal projection analysis, one moves the excitation of projection systems by external energies to a lack of such excitation in these systems. For example, in the profound blackness and darkness of the floatation room there is no visual stimulus coming to the eyes or the visual systems. Similarly in the profound silence there are no sounds coming into the acoustic apparatus, and similarly the other systems are at a very low level of stimulation from the external world.

One might expect then that these systems would appear to be absolutely quiet, dark and empty. This is not so. This is the area in which most subjects begin to get into trouble. It is also the area in which psychiatric and clinical judgments may interfere with the natural development of the phenomena. **In the absence of external excitations coming through the natural end organs the perception systems maintain this activity.** The excitation for this activity comes from other parts of the computer, i.e., from program storage and from internal body sources of excitation. The self-programmer interprets the resultant filling of these perceptual spaces at first *as if* this excitation were coming from outside. In other words, the sources of the excitation are interpreted by the self as if coming from the real world. For certain kinds of persons and personalities this is a very disturbing experience in one sphere or another; for them it is explicable only with telepathy.

We have been taught from babyhood that this kind of phenomena in a totally conscious individual is somehow forbidden, anti-social and possibly even psychotic.

One must analyze this metaprogram that has been implanted in one from childhood, examine its rationality or lack of same and proceed in spite of this kind of an interpretation of the phenomena that occur. Once one has analyzed this as an evasion or a defensive maneuver against seeing the **true state of affairs** one can allow oneself to go on and experience the deeper set of phenomena without interfering with the **natural metaprograms.** After achieving this level of freedom from anxiety, one can then go on to the next stages. (The programming orders for these inner happenings to take place are worked out in advance of the session, at first written down or spoken into a recorder. Later such orders can be programmed without external aids.)

The following phenomenological description has been experienced by one subject under these special conditions. *One experiences an immediate internal reality which is postulated by the self. It is apparent to me that one's own assumptions about this experience generates the whole experience. The experienced affects, the apparent appearance of other persons, the appearance of other beings not human, one's own past phantasies, one's own self-analysis, each can be programmed to happen in interaction with those parts of one's self beyond one's conscious awareness.*

The content experienced under these conditions lacks strong reality clues. *Externally real* displays are not furnished; the excitation from the reality outside does not pattern the displays. Therefore the projections which do occur are from those systems at the next inward level from the operations of the perception apparatus devoted to external reality.

The phenomena that ensue are described by one subject as follows: *the visualization is immersed in darkness in three dimensions at times but only when one evades the emerging* **"multi-dimensional cognitive and conative space."** *One is aware of "the silence" in the hearing sphere; this too gives way to the new space which is developing. The body image fluctuates, appearing and disappearing, as fear or other need builds up. As with the "darkness and the silence" so with the presence or absence of the body image.* Progress in using these projection spaces is measured by one's ability to neither project external reality data from storage into these spaces nor to project into these spaces "the absence of external reality stimuli."

One can project in the visual space living images (external reality equivalents) or blackness (the absence of external reality images). One can project into the acoustic spaces definite sounds, voices, etc. (as if external reality) or one can project *silence* (the absence of sound) in the external reality. One can project the body image also, flexing one's muscles, joints, etc. to reassure oneself the image is functioning with *real feedback* or one can have a primary perception of a *lack of the body image* which is the negative logical alternative to the body image itself.

In each of these dichotomized situations one is *really* projecting external reality and its equivalents (positive or negative). In order to experience the next set of phenomena one must work through these dichotomous symbols of the external world and realize that they are evasions of further penetration to deeper levels.

Once one abandons the use of projection of external reality equivalents from storage, new phenomena appear. **Thought and feeling take over the spaces formerly occupied by external reality equivalents.** (In the older terminology ego expands to fill the subjectively appreciated inner universe.) "Infinity" similar to that in the usual real visual space is also involved and one has the feeling that one's self extends infinitely out in all directions. **The self is still centered at one place but its boundaries have disappeared and it moves out in all directions and extends to fill the limits of the universe as far as one knows them.** The explanation of this phenomenon is that one has merely taken over the perception spaces and filled them with programs, metaprograms, and self-metaprograms which are now modified in the inner perception as if external reality equivalents. This transform, this special mental state, to be appreciated must be experienced directly.

In one's ordinary experience there are dreams which have something of this quality and which show this kind of a phenomenon.

At this level various evasions of realization of what is happening can take place. One can "imagine" that one is traveling through the real universe past suns, galaxies, etc. One can "imagine" that one is communicating with other beings in these other universes.

However, scientifically speaking, it is fairly obvious that one is not doing any of these things and that one's basic beliefs determine what one experiences here. Therefore we say that **the ordinary perception spaces, the ordinary projection spaces, are now filled with cognition and conation processes.** This seems to be a more reasonable point of view to take than the *oceanic feeling,* the *at oneness with the universe* as fusing with Universal Mind as reported in the literature by others for these phenomena. **These states** (or *direct perceptions of reality* as they have been called) **are one's thought and feeling expanding into the circuitry in one's computer usually occupied by perception of external reality in each and every mode,** including vision, audition, proprioception, etc.

A small digression here for purposes of clarifying problems of experiencing these phenomena: In addition to the above discussed factors about fears preventing these phenomena from developing, one must also neutralize various clinical psychiatric explanations and judgments about these phenomena. If one assumes that going through these phenomena is a dangerous procedure in that one might become enamoured of them and hence get into an irreversible *psychosis,* one also can be kept from experiencing these phenomena directly. Since the real necessary and sufficient conditions for the induction of a psychosis are not yet understood, one should not jump to the conclusion that these phenomena themselves are or can cause a psychosis. This has yet to be proven to the satisfaction of everyone in the field. It may be that professional fear is preventing our further analysis of these phenomena. The whole issue of insight into one's own mental processes, the whole issue of self-discipline and inspecting and understanding these processes are at stake here. Those who believe that there is a psychosis impending in all normal people (including professionals) have definite troubles with these kinds of phenomena. Heuristically such beliefs are untenable; such beliefs tend to weaken one's self-discipline under these circumstances and make one rather unfit for such experiences.

A satisfactory analysis of the clinical psychiatric judgments sphere must take place in all trained subjects before proceeding further.

Unless one can move philosophically and scientifically far enough to see the utility of going through these experiences there can be a rapid withdrawal, a faulting out of self from the whole project. One is not willing to undergo the phantasy "dangers" that one sets up ahead of time before going through the experiences. One's fears in this sphere are usually around the questions of whether one will maintain insight into these processes once one has exposed one's self to LSD-25.

Candidly considered one may ask *may not this substance under these conditions change my brain and mind structure irreversibly out of my control?* The proper controls on whether or not there are permanent changes in brains have not been done on animals' nor on humans' brains. So there definitely is a risk in this area. Is one willing to gamble on this particular risk? It is wise to face up to these questions candidly, honestly, and ruthlessly. One is moving into an area which is filled with unknowns of primary importance. The issue of brain and mind injury is a current and important issue which has not been faced by the enthusiasts for LSD-25. It is an issue constantly raised by those who are opposed to the use of LSD-25. The science of finding out whether or not there is any truth in either side (pro or con) is lacking. The pro LSD-group tries to do spectacular things using it. The con-group looks askance at the enthusiasm of the other group and claims that they have lost their insight and are hedonistically over-valuing the effects experienced subjectively. The contra-group tend to claim *brain damage* and/or *mind damage;* the pro-group tends to claim *basic understanding of the mind, a new understanding of mental diseases,* and a *new approach to the psychotherapy of recalcitrant diseases* such as alcoholism. (I leave out here the artistic, religious, and philosophical claims.) (See Leary, Alpert and Metzner, 1964.)

The turning point between the pros and cons of the use of LSD-25 hinges once more philosophically at the edge of this cognitive-conative projection space phenomena: does one lose one's insight and initiative by going here? This question should be asked and answered scientifically and experimentally.

PRACTICAL CONSIDERATIONS

As a pragmatic matter one should do self-analysis in the severely attenuated physical reality without LSD-25 for several exposures before using the substance. One must learn not only to tolerate but to like the experience for several hours at a time. One's fears of the unreleased unconscious programming can be attenuated and analyzed during this period.

Training sessions with LSD-25 with another person must be done before it is combined with the profound physical isolation and solitude. During this period training by the external screens and the projections can be done with doses of LSD-25 from 100 micrograms minimum to the tolerated maximum of that individual. During this period one must face the fears of LSD-25 itself and the fears mentioned above of damage to one's brain and one's mind by this agent. One must also face the hedonistic, narcissistic pleasure induction and maintenance possible with LSD-25, and one must make one's own decision about how to handle these pleasures versus those which are brought about in the external reality.

In the profound physical isolation situation one acquires, or one has, or one develops a confidence in one's body to function quite automatically and to take care of itself. The whole problem of air supply, keeping one's face above the water, the action of respiration and of heart, etc., are all turned over to the proto-human survival programs to maintain themselves. All tendencies on the part of a subject to control or to monitor his own respiration or his own heart action should be discouraged. The same applies to the gastrointestinal tract and the genitourinary tract. Insofar as can be achieved automatic operations of these systems should be encouraged. Gradually they will assume their proper low-level expression in the psychic life of the individual subject. Confidence in their continued operation without attention by one's self (by the self-metaprograms) can be achieved. These considerations are particularly important with the LSD-25 as the physical isolation and solitude begin to develop.

On the analytic side one must have analyzed and dealt with one's unconscious death wishes. Up to a certain critical point one knows and feels the probability of survival under conditions over which one has control. One has already experienced internal mechanisms which may have tried to take over and deal a death-seeking blow to one. This kind of material must have been thoroughly analyzed with an external analyst before one approaches experiments such as these. One's self and one's analyst must be content that the level of control of such internal mechanisms is such that the probability of their dealing a death-seeking blow is low enough to risk exposure to these new conditions. This point cannot be emphasized strongly enough. Those who are acquainted with the phenomena during classical psychoanalysis realize that certain kinds of personalities and certain individuals during analysis and after analysis can go through depressive phases in which such death wishes can be acted out. **The seeds of destruction of self can be buried in the deeper metaprograms and programs of one's own computer. Certain kinds of neuronal activities can destroy an organism.** These are the kinds of activities which one must know and be aware of the signs and the symbols of evocation of these systems within one's self.

Such negative phenomena are usually seen after the first session or two with LSD-25. The residual unanalyzed portion of these programs are usually projected and acted out as a consequence of their release by this agent. Several analytic sessions with an external analyst are thus necessary for maximum safety and minimum risk in these experiments.

In the farthest and deepest state of isolation, one's basic needs and one's assumptions about self become evident. The existence of self and one's belief in the existence of one's self are made manifest. The positive or negative sign of values that one places upon one's self and upon the existence of one's self begins to show its force and strength. The problems discussed, but generally unfaced in a religious context in the external real world, are faced and can be *lived out* with a freedom unavailable since childhood.

The problem of the dissolution of one's conscious self by death of the body is studiable. One's evasions of this problem and of facing it can be projected into studiable areas of one's experience. The existence theorem for spiritual and psychic entities is also testable and the strength of one's belief in these entities can be analyzed. Evasions of self-analysis and evasions of taking on certain kinds of beliefs can be tested.

In this area the denial and negation mechanisms of classical psychoanalysis show their strength. Previous analysis can train one to recognize that when data cannot be called up or when displays cannot be constructed or when certain operations cannot be carried out, one can see the cause currently existing. The set of inhibitory and repressive devices in one's computer is hard at work. In such inhibitory and repressive states preprogrammed sets of basic assumptions to be explored are incompletely carried out. One quickly finds areas of the consequences of the assumed beliefs, which one cannot enter or only enters with fear, with anger, or with love, carried over from some other programming.

DEFINITION OF A GENERAL PURPOSE
SELF-METAPROGRAM

The essential features and the goals sought in the self-analysis are in the metaprogram: *make the computer general purpose*. In this sense we mean that in the general purpose nature of the computer there can be no display, no acting, nor an ideal which is forbidden to a consciously-willed metaprogram. Nor is any display, acting or ideal made without being consciously meta-programmed. In each case of course one is up against the limits of the unique computer which is one's own. There are certain kinds of metaprograms, displays, acting, or ideals which are beyond the capacity of a particular computer. However, one's imagined limits are sometimes smaller than those which one can achieve with special work. The metaprogram of the specific beliefs about the limits of one's self are at stake here. One's ability to achieve certain special states of consciousness, for example, are generally preprogrammed by basic beliefs taken on in childhood. If the computer is to maintain its general purpose nature (which presumably was there in childhood), one must recapture a far greater range of phenomena than one expects that one has available. For instance, one should be able to program in practically any area possible within human imagination, human action or human being.

As explorations deepen, one can see the evading nature of many programs which one previously considered basic to one's private and professional philosophy. As one opens up the depths, it is wise not to privately or publicly espouse as *ultimate* any *truths* one *finds* in the following areas: the universe in general, beings not human, thought transference, life after death, transmigration of souls, racial memories, species-jumping-thinking, non-physical action at a distance, and so forth. Such ideas may merely be a reflection of one's needs in terms of one's own survival. **Ruthless self-analysis as to one's needs for certain kinds** of ideas in these areas must be explored honestly and truthfully. The rewarding- and positively-reinforcing effects of LSD-25 must be remembered and emphasized; one overvalues the results of one's chemically rewarding thinking.

Once one has done such deep analysis one later finds deeper that these needs were generating these ideas. One's public need to proclaim them to one's self and to others, as if they are the ultimate truth, is an expression of one's need to believe. Insight into the fact that one is enthused because the positive, start-and-maintain, rewarding sign has been chemically stamped on these ideas must be remembered.

An explorer operating at these depths cannot afford such childish baggage. These are disguises of and evasions of the ultimate dissolution of self; the maintenance of pleasure and of life are insisting on denial of death. If one stops at these beliefs, no progress in further analysis can be made. These beliefs are *analysis dissolvers*. One might call these lazy assumptions which prevent one from pushing deeper into self and avoid expending any great effort in this deeper direction. One of these very powerful evasions is an hedonistic acceptance of things as they are with conversion of most of them to a pleasant glow. Another similar evasion is deferring discussion of such basic issues until one's *life after death*.

A possibly great spur to work in this area for certain kinds of persons is the acceptance of unknowables and of the unknown itself. A powerful wish to push into the unknown further than those ahead of one in calendar time is helpful in terms of one's motivation at this point. Everyone has his say about the truth in this area. Many other persons would like very much to have one follow their metaprograms. In my own view I would prefer to be a questing mind reporting on some interesting journeys. Insofar as I fail to be this, I, too, am guilty of attempting to metaprogram the reader.

In summary then one starts on the deeper journeys, independently, metaprogrammed properly, and relatively safe but without evasions. After having been through some of the innermost depths of self, a result is that they are only one's own beliefs and their multitudes of randomized logical consequences deep down inside one's self. There is nothing else but stored experience.

2

Summary of Experiments
in Self-Metaprogramming with
LSD-25

In order to test the validity of some of the basic assumptions implicit in the theory of the human computer, a series of experiments were designed and carried out in the LSD-25 state, in physical isolation, and solitude. One point of primary interest during these experiments was to find out what level of intensity of belief in a set of assumptions could be achieved. The assumptions tested in this set of experiments are not those of current science: they are not in the conscious working repertory of this scientist; nor were they consciously acceptable to him.

In this short account it is not intended to give all of the details of either the self-metaprogramming language that was used or the details of the elicited phenomena. The account is purposely sparse, condensed, and compressed. Abstracted from the complexity of the totality of the experiments and their results are only those *formal* descriptions which may serve as guide posts to others attempting to reproduce these or similar experiments. It is not intended to complicate this account with the personal aspects of the metaprogramming, the elicited phenomena, or difficulties encountered. For those researchers who are interested in this work's reproduction in themselves, these assumptions (or similar ones) and these results can be translated into their own metaprogramming language and such workers can obtain their unique results.

To claim validity of details beyond myself is not my aim. There probably are those men who are prepared well enough to attempt reproducing what has been done here in themselves. The descriptions are given so that the sources of the human computer theory are available to professionals.

This particular set of existence theorems is selected for experiment for a number of reasons. There are a number of persons (Blum, 1964) who experimented with the LSD-25 state who write as if they believe implicitly in the objective reality of causes outside themselves for certain kinds of experiences undergone with these particular beliefs.

I do not think it wise to espouse either the existence or the non-existence theorem for this set of basic supra-self-metaprograms (Fig. 1). **To become impartial, dispassionate, and *general purpose*, objective, and open-ended, one must test and adjust the level of credence in each of his sets of beliefs.** If ever Man is to be faced with real organisms with greater wisdom, greater intellect, greater minds than any single man has, then we must be open, unbiased, sensitive, general purpose, and dispassionate. Our needs for phantasies must have been analyzed and seen for what they are and are not or we will be in even graver troubles than we are today.

Our search for mentally healthy paths to human progress in the innermost realities depends upon progress in this area. Many men have floundered in this area of belief: I hope this work can help to find a way through one of our stickiest intellectual-emotional regions.

Most of these beliefs are ones which have been abandoned in the fields of endeavor called science. Such beliefs continue to be found in the field known as religion. Some of these beliefs are labeled in modern psychiatric medicine and anthropology as *superstitions, psychotic beliefs,* etc. Other persons present these beliefs in the writings called *science fiction*.

This set of basic postulates (or beliefs) is conceived and used to program several sessions with LSD-25 plus physical isolation in solitude. Above all these metaprograms to be experimented upon is one metaprogram of value to this subject: his overall policy is the intent to explore, to observe, to analyze. Hence there is an important additional **basic metaprogram**: *analyze self to understand one's thinking and true motives more thoroughly.* This is the conscious motivational strategy. At times this metaprogram dominates the scene, at times others do. The resolve exists, however, to generate a net effect with this instruction uppermost in the computer hierarchy.

EXPERIMENTS ON BASIC METAPROGRAMS OF EXISTENCE

Preliminary to the experiments in changing basic beliefs, many experiments with the profound physical isolation and solitude situation were carried out over a period of several years. These experiences were followed by combining the LSD-25 state and the physical isolation state in a second period of several years. The minimum time between experiments was thirty days, the maximum time several months. [Tables 1, 7 and 8]

Basic Belief No. 1
Basic Belief No. 1 was made possible by the early isolation results: *Assume that the subject's body and brain can operate comfortably isolated without him paying any attention to it.* This belief expresses the faith that one has in one's experience in the isolation situation, that one can consciously ignore the necessities of breathing and other bodily functions, and that they will take care of themselves automatically without detailed attention on the part of one's self. This result allowed **existence** metaprograms to be made in relative safety.

Successful *leaving of the body and parking it* in isolation for **periods of twenty minutes to two hours were successful** in sixteen different experiments. This success, in turn, allowed other basic beliefs to be experimented upon. The basic belief that one could **leave the body and explore new universes** was successfully programmed in the first eight different experiments lasting from five minutes to forty minutes; the later eight experiments were on the *cognitional multidimensional space* without the *leaving the body* metaprogram (see previous section on Projection for the *cognition space* phenomenon).

Basic Belief No. 2

The subject sought *beings other than himself, not human, in whom he existed and who control him and other human beings.* Thus the subject found whole new *universes* containing great varieties of *beings*, some greater than himself, some equal to himself, and some lesser than himself.

Those greater than himself were a set which was so huge in space-time as to make the subject feel *as a mere mote in their sunbeam, a single microflash of energy in their time scale, my forty-five years are but an instant in their lifetime, a single thought in their vast computer, a mere particle in their assemblages of living cognitive units.* He felt he was in the absolute unconsicous of these beings. He experienced many more sets all so much greater than himself that they were almost inconceivable in their complexity, size and time scales.

Those *beings* which were close to the subject in complexity-size-time were dichotomized into *the evil ones* and *the good ones.* The *evil* ones (subject said) were busy with purposes so foreign to his own that he had many near-misses and almost fatal accidents in encounters with them; they were almost totally unaware of his existence and hence almost wiped him out, apparently without knowing it. The subject says that the *good* ones *thought good thoughts to him, through him, and to one another.* They were at least conceivably human and humane. He interpreted them as alien yet *friendly*. They were not so alien as to be completely removed from human beings in regard to their purposes and activities.

Some of these beings (the subject reported) are programming us in the long term. They nurture us. They experiment on us. They control the probability of our discovering and exploiting new science. He reports that discoveries such as nuclear energy, LSD-25, RNA-DNA, etc., are under probability control by these beings. Further, humans are tested by some of these beings and cared for by others. Some of them have programs which include our survival and progress. Others have programs which include oppositions to these *good* programs and include our ultimate demise as a species. Thus the subject interpreted the evil ones as willing to sacrifice us in their experiments; hence they are *alien and removed from us*. The subject reported with this set of beliefs that *only limited choices are still available to us as a species. We are an ant colony in their laboratory.*

Basic Belief No. 3

The subject assumed **the existence of beings in whom humans exist and who directly control humans.** This is a tighter control program than the previous one and assumes continuous day and night, second to second, control, as if each human being were a cell in a larger organism. Such beings insist upon activities in each human being totally under the control of the organism of which each human being is a part. In this state there is no free will and no freedom for an individual. This supra-self-metaprogram was entered twice by the subject; each time he had to leave it; for him it was too anxiety-provoking. In the first case he *became a part of a vast computer in which he was one element.* In the second case he was *a thought in a much larger mind: being modified rapidly, flexibly and plastically.*

All of the above experiments were done looking upward in Fig. 1 from the self-programmer to the supra-self-metaprograms. A converse set of experiments was done in which the self-metaprogrammer looked downward towards the metaprograms, the programs and the lower levels of Fig. 1.

Basic Belief No. 4

One set of basic beliefs can be subsumed under the directions *seek those beings whom we control and who exist in us.* With this program the subject found old models in himself (old programs, old metaprograms, implanted by others, implanted by self, injected by parents, by teachers, etc.). He found that these were disparate and separate autonomous *beings* in himself. He described them as a *noisy group*. His incorporated parents, his siblings, his own offspring, his teachers, his wife seemed to be a disorganized crowd within him, each running and arguing a program with him and in him. While he watched, battles took place between these *models* during the experiment. **He settled many disparate and nonintegrated points between these *beings* and gradually incorporated more of them into the self-metaprogram.**

After many weeks of self-analysis outside the experimental milieu (and some help with his former analyst), it was seen that these *beings within the self* were also those other *beings outside self* of the other experiments. The subject described the projected as-if-outside beings to be *cognitional carnivores attempting to eat up his self-metaprogram and wrest control from him.* As the various levels of metaprograms became straightened out in the subject, he was able to categorize and begin to control the various levels as they were presented during these experiments. As his apparently unconscious needs for credence in these beliefs were attenuated with analytic work, his freedom to move from one set of basic beliefs to another was increased and the anxiety associated with this kind of movement gradually disappeared.

A basic overall metaprogram was finally generated: For his own intellectual satisfaction the **subject found that he best assume that all of the phenomena that took place existed only in his own brain and in his own mind. Other assumptions about the** existence of these *beings* had become subjects suitable for research rather than subjects for blind (unconscious, conscious) *belief* for this person.

Basic Belief No. 5

Experiments also were done upon **movements of self forward and back in space-time.** The results showed that when attempting to go *forward into the future* the subject began to *realize* his own goals for that future, and imagine *wishful thinking solutions* to current problems. When he put in the metaprogram for going back into his own childhood, *real and phantasy memories* were evoked and integrated. When he pushed back through to the **in utero** situation, he found an early nightmare which was reinvoked and solved. Relying on his scientific *knowledge*, he pushed the program back through previous generations, prehuman primates, carnivores, fish and protozoa. He experienced a *sperm-egg explosion* on the way through this past *reinvocation* of *imaginary* experience.

The last set of experiments (see **Use of Projection** section) was made possible by the results of the previous set. Progress in controlling the projection metaprogram resulted from the *other universes* experiments. Finally the subject understood and had become familiar with his need for *phantasied other universes.* Analytic work allowed him to bypass this need and penetrate into the *cognitional multidimensional projection spaces.* **Experiments in programming in this *innermost space* showed results quite satisfying to a high degree of credence in the belief that all experiments in the series showed inner happenings without needing *the participation of outer causes.*** The need for the constant use of *outer causes* was found to be a projected outward metaprogram to avoid taking personal responsibility for portions of the contents of his own mind. His dislike for certain kinds of his own nonsensical programs caused him to project them and thus avoid admitting they were his.

In summation, the subjectively apparent results of the experiments were to straighten out a good deal of the "nonsense" in this subject's computer. Through these experiments he was able to examine some *warded-off beliefs and defensive structures* accumulated throughout his life. The net result was a feeling of greater integration of self and a feeling of positive affect for the current structure of himself, combined with an improved **skepticism of the validity of subjective judging of events in self.**

Some *objective* testing of these essentially subjective judgments have been initiated through cooperation with other persons. Such objective testing is very difficult; this area needs a great deal of future research work. We need better investigative techniques, combining subjective and behavioral (verbal) techniques. The major feeling that one has after such experiences and experiments is that the fluidity and plasticity of one's computer has certain limits to it, and that those limits have been enlarged somewhat by the experiments. How long such enlargement lasts and to what extent are still not known of course. A certain amount of continued critical skepticism about and in the self-metaprogram (and in its *felt* changes) is very necessary for a scientist exploring these areas.

METAPROGRAMMATIC RESULTS OF
BELIEF EXPERIMENTS

The metatheoretical consideration of these experiments and the results are as follows: One supra-metaprogrammatic assumption about these experiments is the formalistic view of the origins of mathematics and of thinking. As was said in the preface, at one extreme of the organization of human thinking is the *formal logical basic assumption* set of metatheories. These experiments were done with this view in mind and the results were interpreted from this point of view.

Obviously this point of view does not test the "objective"

validity of the experiences. It merely assumes that, if one plugs the proper beliefs into the metaprogrammatic levels of the computer that, the computer will then construct (from the myriads of elements in memory) those possible *experiences* that fit this particular set of rules. Those programs will be run off and those displays made, which are appropriate to the basic assumptions and their stored programming.

Another way of looking at the results and at the metaprogramming is that we start out with a basic set of beliefs, believe them to be "objectively" valid (not just "formally" valid) and do the experiments and interpret them with this point of view. If one proceeds along these lines, one can quickly reach the end of one's ability to interpret the results. One finds that one cannot grasp conceptually the phenomena that ensue. With this metatheory, this type of experience is not just the computer operating in isolation, confinement and solitude on preprogrammed material being elicited from memory, but is *really in communication with other beings, and the influence on one's self by them is real.*

Thus in this case one is assuming the existence theorem in regard to the basic assumptions, i.e., there is objective validity to them quite outside of self and one's making the assumptions. This epistemological position can also be investigated by these methods. This is somewhat the position that was taken by Aldous Huxley and by various other groups. For example, pursuit of certain non-Western philosophies as the *Ultimate Truth* was generated by these persons.

One cannot take sides on these two widely diverse epistemological bases. On the one hand we have the basic assumptions of the modern scientists and on the other hand the basic assumptions of those interested in the *religious* aspect of existence. If one is to remain philosophic and objective in this field, one must dispassionately survey both of these extreme metatheoretical positions.

One basic lesson learned from these experiments is that, in general, one's preferences for various kinds of metatheoretical positions are dictated by considerations other than one's ideals of impartiality, objectivity, and a dispassionate view. The metatheoretical position held by scientists in general is espoused for purposes of defining *the truth*, for purposes of understanding in their particular compartment of science, for acceptance among other scientists and for each one's own *internal security operations* with respect to his own unconscious programs. It is to be expected that anxiety is engendered in some scientists by making the above assumptions *as if true* (even temporarily) in an experimental framework. One can easily be panicked by the invasion of the self-metaprograms by automatic *existence* programs from below the level of one's awareness, programs which may strike at the existence of self, at the control of self, at the origins of self, at the destinations of self, and of the relations of self to a known external reality.

Possibly one of the **safest** positions to take with regard to all of these phenomena is that given in this paper, i.e., the formalistic view in which one makes the assumption that the computer itself generates all of the phenomena experienced. This is an acceptable assumption of modern science. This is the so-called *common sense* assumption. This is the assumption acceptable to one's colleagues in science.

Such considerations, of course, do not touch upon nor prove the validity or invalidity of the assumptions nor of the results of the experiments. In order to leave this theory open-ended and to allow for the presence of the unknown, it is necessary to take the ontological and epistemological position that **one cannot know as a result of this kind of solitudinous experiment whether or not the phenomena are explicable only by non-biocomputer interventions or only by happenings within the computer itself, or both.**

I wish to emphasize that there is a necessity not to espouse *a truth* because it is safe. **Being driven to a set of assumptions because one is afraid of another set and their consequences is the most passionate and nonobjective kind of philosophy.** Too many intellectuals and scientists (almost unconsciously) use basic assumptions as defenses against their fears of other assumptions and their consequences. Until we can train ourselves to be dispassionate and accept both the assumptions and the results of making them without arrogance, without pride, without misplaced enthusiasm, without fear, without panic, without anger, hence without emotional involvement in the results or in the theories, we cannot advance this *inner* science of Man very far.

Those who wish to embrace the *truth* of an alternative set of assumptions as an escape from the basic assumptions of modern science are equally at fault. Those who must find *a communication with other beings* in this kind of experiment will **apparently** find it. One must be aware that there are (as in the child) needs within one's self for finding certain kinds of phenomena and espousing them as the ultimate truth. Such childlike needs dictate their own metaprograms.

I am not agreeing with any extreme group in interpreting these results. It is convenient for me to assume, as of this time, that these phenomena all occurred within the biocomputer. I tend to assume that ESP cannot have played a role. At the moment this is the position which I find to be most tenable in a logical sense. I do not wish to be dogmatic about this. I wish to indicate that this is where I stand as of the writing describing this particular stage of the work. I await demonstrations of the validity of alternative existence theorems.

If ever good, hard-nosed, common sense, unequivocal evidence for the existence of currently unaccepted assumptions is presented by those who have thoroughly attenuated their childish needs for particular beliefs, I hope I am prepared to examine it dispassionately and thoroughly. The pitfalls of group interlock are quite as insidious as the pitfalls of one's own phantasizing.

Group acceptance of undemonstrated existence theorems and of seductive beliefs adds no more validity to the theorems and to the beliefs than one's own phantasizing can add. Anaclitic group behavior is no better than solitudinous phantasies of *the truth*. Where *agreed-upon* truth can exist in the science of the innermost realities is not and cannot yet be settled. Beginnings have been made by many men, satisfying proofs by one.

¤ 3
Personal Metaprogrammatic Language:
An Example of Its Properties

Among all of the languages possessed by one's self some are used to control the metaprogrammatic level in Fig. 1. The self-metaprogrammer exerts control through **the personal metaprogrammatic language.** This is the language which controls the computer itself, how it operates, and how it computes as an integral whole. **Each human computer has a unique private control language in its unique stored programs, stored metaprograms, and stored self-metaprograms.** This language is not all shared in the usual public domain of the language acquired in childhood.

In this particular instance one can visualize in Fig. 1 certain levels in and at which the experiments were done in detail. This **control language and control of the biocomputer itself can be changed as new understanding of control allows new control.** This *language* has aspects which are nonverbal, nonvocal and can be more emotional and/or mathematical than they are linguistic. Here we are expressing some "linguistic" aspects and some of the "mathematical" nonverbal experiences. We are limited in this public expression to the consensus non-private language.

The experiments were designed along the lines of finding solutions to certain personal problems within the biocomputer. These problems are the basic ones of the presence of antithetical and contradictory metaprograms. In Fig. 1 some of these paradoxical and agonistic problems appear at the supra-self-metaprogram level and some at the metaprogram level. One such experiment was on a spontaneous occurrence of a phrase (during the LSD-25 state) which took on elements of humor and the aspect *as if a great discovery.* The private metaprogrammatic control instruction is: *the key is no key.*

In the external reality, stimulus for this statement was a number of keys which the subject had been carrying around for several years. He suddenly became aware that he had in his life many locks. Thus it was necessary for him to carry many keys. At times these keys were felt as a physical and a mental burden which slowed the efficient operation of his life. These were aspects of the phrase *key* which were real keys, real locks on real doors to real rooms, real houses, real offices, etc. At that particular moment this seemed to be the epitome of modern civilization: to have doors, to have locks on those doors, and have privileged persons who possessed the keys to open those doors.

The subject next moved from the meanings in the *external reality metaprogram* to another level in which he internalized this picture of the door, the room, the lock, the key. He visualized his own antithetical metaprograms as existing in rooms separated by doors which had locks on them. He was searching for the keys to open the doors.

As these inner *rooms* (categories, problems, antitheses) became embodied in the *locked door* imagined-projected metaphor the subject began to walk through metaprogrammatic storage looking for a key to open the next door into the further recesses of the rooms. As he moved he began to see that the doors were defined as doors by his own computer; locks were defined as locks; and that keys were defined as necessary to open the locks.

In a moment of insight, he saw that the defined boundaries (the doors, the walls, ceilings, the floors, and the locks themselves and their keys) were a convenient metaprogram dividing up his knowledge and his control mechanisms into compartments in an *artificial personal* fashion.

He explored many rooms with many different kinds of knowledge in the rooms. The walls slowly began to dissolve, some of them melted and flowed away; other rooms were revealed as solid and the doors with secure locks rather numerous; some keys were missing.

Most of the hypothesized *building* inside his own mind, however, now became open spaces with information freely available without the former walls between arbitrary *rooms of categories.* Those rooms, locks, and keys that were left were quite basic to the development of this individual's self-metaprogram.

Some of these *rooms* were created in childhood in response to situations over which the self-metaprogrammer had no control. These rooms housed ideas and systems of thinking which to this particular subject evoked intense fear or intense anger as he approached with the intent of opening the doors. The locks did not respond to frontal assaults. These rooms turned out to be very difficult to define out of existence in order to have their contents interact with the rest of the metaprogrammatic level.

The subject underwent a frantic and frightened search for the keys to the locks of these *strong-rooms.* He became alternately fearful and angry. He made several assaults on walls, doors, ceilings and floors of these closed rooms without much success.

He went away from these rooms into *other universes and other spaces* and left the computer to work out solutions below his levels of awareness.

Later with higher motivational energy the subject returned to the problem of the lock, the doors and the rooms somewhat refreshed by the experiences in the other realms.

Mathematical transformations were next tried in the approach to the locked rooms. The concept of the key fitting into the lock and the necessity of finding the key were abandoned and the rooms were approached as *topological puzzles.* In the multidimensional cognitional and visual space the rooms were now manipulated without the necessity of the key in the lock.

Using the transitional concept that the lock is a hole in the door through which one can exert an effort for a topological transformation, one could turn the room into another topological form other than a closed box. The room in effect was turned inside out through the hole, through the lock leaving the contents outside and the room now a collapsed balloon placed farther from the self-metaprogrammer. Room after room was thus defined as turned inside out with the contents spewed forth for use by the self-metaprogrammer. Once this control *key* worked, it continued automatically to its own limits.

With this sort of an "intellectual crutch," as it were, entire new areas of basic beliefs were entered upon. Most of the rooms which before had appeared as strong rooms with big powerful walls, doors, and locks now ended up as empty balloons. The greatly defended contents of the rooms in many cases turned out to be relatively trivial programs and episodes from childhood which had been over-generalized and over-valued by this particular human computer. **The devaluation** of the general purpose properties of the human biocomputer was one such room. In childhood the many episodes which led to the self-metaprogrammer not remaining general purpose but becoming more and more limited and *specialized* were entered upon. Several layers of the supra-self-metaprograms laid down in childhood were opened up.

The mathematical operation which took place in the computer was the movement of energies and masses of data from the supra-self-metaprogram down to the self-metaprogrammatic level and below. At the same time there was the knowledge that programmatic materials had been moved from the *supra-self-position* to the *under-self-controlled position* at the programmatic level. These operations were all filed in metaprogram storage under the title "The key is no key."

It was noticed that the necessity for locks and for keys in the real world had to be dealt with. There was an interval of time in which the subject was quite willing to throw all of his keys away and keep all of the real doors of his life unlocked. That was tried briefly and resulted in a theft. This immediately brought home the obvious fact that the external reality programs cannot be controlled by the self-metaprogram. There are other human bio-computers and a real external reality which has unpredictable properties not under the control of the self-metaprogrammer. Therefore there must remain in the supra-self-metaprogram certain rules for conduct of the human computer in the external reality. There must remain a certain modicum of real supra-self control and respect for the external reality's part of the supra-self-metaprogram.

As it was stated elsewhere (Lilly, 1956, Lilly and Shurley, 1960): *the province of the mind is the only area of science in which what one believes to be true either is true or becomes true within limits to be determined experimentally.* This particular subject saw that *the key is no key* is a private self-metaprogramming language phrase and should not be applied to the external reality metaprogram nor should it be applied to other human biocomputers (at least without careful consideration of their capabilities and their own supra-self-metaprograms). As it were similar topological transformations under control of the self-metaprogrammer may not yet have developed within the given other person. The kinds of phenomena expressed by this unique private human computer (*The key is no key*) may be totally inapplicable to others.

Metatheoretically considered, however, the above operation can be re-expressed by a given individual and elaborated and differentiated along other coordinates. For those willing to try these experiments I wish to add a suggestion: It is necessary to explore all aspects of one's body image, one's childish emotional regions, one's real body in various states and with special stimuli in addition to those from the body itself. With such explorative training one can do topological transformations which can result in step-wise changes in metaprogramming and in metaprograms themselves. **Bias, prejudice, preconception and intransigence in explicit areas are seen as supra-self-metaprograms which are inappropriate.** Until there can be highly motivated mathematical transformations within the areas of control metaprograms, major changes are not made.

The above all-too-condensed summary of these experiments and their results illustrates the linguistic symbolization of mathematical operations; this operation offers a certain kind of shorthand to the human computer. **Linguistic symbols can be used for storing symbols which represent whole areas of operations in the computer.** *The key is no key* is a version of the actual operations which it symbolizes. The statement is in the language of the child as the young computer originally stored it. The actual operations taking place in the adult symbolized by *the key is no key* are a complex rendering of more advanced ideas, some of which are circuit-like, some of which are topological transformations and some of which are in multidimensional matrices.

A given human computer is limited in its operations by its own acquired mathematical conceptual machinery; this is part of its supra-self-metaprograms. Maximum control over the metaprogrammatic level by the self-metaprogram is achieved not by direct "one to one" orders and instructions from the one level to the other. **The control is based upon exploration of n-dimensional spaces and finding key points for transformations, first in decisive small local regions which can result in large-scale transformations.** (This modeling reminds one of Ashby's *Design for a Brain*, 1954, in which a large "homeostat" stimulated in one small region makes large adjustments throughout itself in order to compensate for the small change.)

One key in the mind is to hunt for those discontinuities in the structure of the thinking which reveal a critical turn-over point at which one can exert emotional energy so as to cause a transformation in all of that region.

The analogy of the *key in the lock* is part of this subject's human computer as a child. The *lock* is now transformed into an n-dimensional choice-point at which one could exert the proper amount of energy in the proper dimensions and in proper directions in those dimensions and find a radical transformation of all the metaprograms in that region of the computer. In a three-dimensional *geometrical* model of such operations (in which one decreases the number of dimensions so that they can be visualized in visual space) one can think of oddly-shaped *rubber* surfaces connected on lines, on points and over large areas which are inflated to different amounts and differing pressures so as to fill a very large room. These membranes are of different colors and various regions are differently lighted and the whole is considered to be pulsing and changing shapes but not changing contact between surfaces, lines, or points. One can imagine one's self moving through these complex surfaces. There are various colors lighted from various directions. One hunts for that zone in which one can exert maximum amount of effect in terms of the redistribution of bond energies, over point, line, and surface areas of contact. One may also exert the maximum effect on the differential pressures in the spaces bounded by each of the surfaces where closed.

After sufficient study of this model one discovers that the points of contact between the membranes are not as fixed as when first seen. What one saw at first was a frozen instant of time extending over a long period of time as if the model were static. Suddenly one realizes that the points of contact are the sharing of portions of these surfaces along appropriate lines at given instants and that these boundaries are changing constantly. One suddenly also discovers that the colors are moving over the surfaces and passing the boundaries. This particular model is a small region in a larger universe filled with such surfaces and intersections and spaces between. One also discovers that the light sources are within certain of these sheets shining through to others and that the hue and intensity are varying according to some local rules.

One moves away from the model and sees that it is filling a *universe*; one moves back into the model and begins to look carefully at one thin membrane. As the structure of the membrane is revealed and the structure of the intersection between the membrane is seen, it turns out that there is microcircuitry within the membrane at a molecular and atomic level. There are energies moving in prescribed paths (sometimes in a noisy fashion) in multiple directions within the membrane. At the intersections collisions occur (electrons, mesons, protons, neutrons, neutrinos, etc. are moving from one sheet to the other in both directions). Sheets that are immediately adjacent are seen to be doing local computations at very high speed. The intersections are now seen as micromolecular-atomic switch lines, switch surfaces, and switch points.

Thus one finds that the phrase *The key is no key* has grown into a new conception of a computer. This computer within itself ideally recognizes no locks, no forbidden transitions, no areas in which data cannot be freely moved from one zone to another. At the boundaries of the computer, however, there are still, as it were *categorical imperatives*. Now the problem becomes not the boundaries within the computer but the boundaries outside it. By *outside* I do not mean only the integumentary boundaries of the real body. I mean other sources of influence than through the bottom layer of the external chemical physical reality (Fig. 1). To symbolize this doubt, this skepticism, about the boundaries of the computer and the influences that can be brought to bear upon them other than those coming through the physical-chemical reality, a line is placed above the supra-self-metaprograms and is labeled *unknown* (Fig. 1).

In the mind of this subject the unknown must take precedence. It is placed above the supra-self-metaprogram because it contains some of the goals of this particular human computer. **This exploration of the inner reality presupposes that the inner reality contains large unknowns which are worth exploring. However, to explore them it is necessary (1) to recognize their existence and (2) to prepare one's computer for the exploration.** If one is to explore the *unknown* one should take the minimum amount of baggage and not load one's self down with conceptual machinery which cannot be flexibly reoriented to accept and investigate the *unknown*. The next stage of development of those who have the courage and the necessary inner apparatus to do it, is exploration in depth of this vast *inner unknown* region. For this task we need the best kind of thinking of which man is capable. We dissolve and/or reprogram the doctrinaire and ideological approaches to these questions.

To remain skeptical of even this formalization of this particular human computer's approach to this region is desirable. One does not over-value this particular approach; one looks for alternative approaches for exploratory purposes. Freedom from the tyranny of the supra-self-metaprograms is sought but not to the point at which other human computers control this particular human computer. Deep and basic interlock between selected human computers is needed for this exploration. Conceptualization of the thinking machine itself is needed by the best minds available for this task. In a sense, we create the explorers in this area.

4

Metaprogramming in the Presence of a
Fixed Neurological Program (Migraine):
Example of Perception and Belief
Interactions

Specific example is given: some experiments were done on reprogramming a specific biocomputer (migraine case) in the LSD-25 state.

Under certain special circumstances it has been found possible to program certain trends in perception and project them into the visual space for study. Among such processes are *the apparent presence of other persons*. One's belief in the reality of of these *presences* is not at stake here. Unless one purposely intensifies the belief in the reality of these presences, one can detect that they are not *existing in the external reality*. The safe metaprogram to use is that they exist only in the mind even though they appear to exist outside the body.

One may ask the question: do these programs exist continuously below the threshold of consciousness in the usual mental state, or are they created **de novo** in or by the LSD-25 state? Current psychoanalytic and psychiatric theories state that they exist in the "unconscious" below the levels of awareness and are evoked from that region of the computer by the LSD-25 state. All we can say here is that this looks like the more likely of the two alternatives; however, the other one should be kept in mind. Some of these below-threshold-programs once detected with the LSD-25 state can (in solitude without LSD-25) be just detected near threshold in a highly motivated state. Without LSD-25 one can achieve the necessary excitation of these programs to force them above threshold.

In one particular subject migraine was used as an advantageous *tracer* and a spur to the self-analysis. In this case there were asymmetries of the spatial perception fields. The right side of the visual field was very different from the left side. (What was seen from the right eye was different from that seen with the left eye.) These differences reside in color, in the persistence of after-images, in the occurrences of scotoma during a migraine attack, etc. (As is well known in the clinical literature such conditions can exist easily forty years or more.) Among these asymmetries there are spatial distortions of the visual system. In this particular case the right eye is more sensitive, has a lower threshold for photophobia and pain in general. The sensations and skin perceptions on the right side of the head are less pleasant and stronger than those on the left. The migraine attack is confined to the right side of the head.

At times correct programming can be achieved in the LSD-25 state so that these cephalic differences can be enhanced, studied, and projected. Recall and living out of past experiences from childhood show a traumatic use of the right side of the head. In the LSD-25 state abrupt physical blows to the right side of the head with violent shrinking away from the source, with right eye closure falling away to the left, and brief apparent "loss of consciousness" was experienced. This is an example of a *long-term (apparently) built-in unconscious program.* This experience was not elicited without the help of the LSD-25 state nor without the help of abreactions in classical psychoanalysis. All that can be seen of this program during the usual daily e.r. state is the asymmetry of perception.

In the LSD-25 state this autonomous program generated some *presences not real but perceived as if real.* When with proper metaprogramming this effect was raised above threshold, the *presences* were felt and seen as shadowy creatures or persons coming in from the right side of the visual field out of darkness. The impression is that the spatial field of perception becomes distorted in such a way that the presences can penetrate the distorted field.

In thinking about this effect the patient generated a theory of the projections *as if it was no projection.* The patient states that these are *beings from another dimension penetrating through a hole between their and our universes.* (This attribution of causes makes no sense unless it is believed implicitly.) Once the intensity of belief in this system is lowered, the critical threshold for the distortion of the perceptual field becomes obvious and the unconsciously programmed projection process becomes detectable. The artificial beings now are no longer that, they are merely distortions of the visual field because of some peculiar development of the nervous system. The dramatic bringing in of *external beings* was shown to have a need of its own, a relief from the solitude and isolation. Essential loneliness gives rise to the creation of those beings within this particular person. The necessity of projecting his own anger and fears by the creation of these *beings* was found in the subsequent analysis.

After these experiences study of these phenomena without LSD-25 in solitude and isolation showed that the distorted field can be detected by relaxation of vigilance and by free association into the edges of the perceptual spaces using any random sequence of stimuli for the projection energy. Without the LSD-25 the *beings or presences* do not appear. Peculiar distortions of the perceptual space do appear. These distortions gave the excuse for the projection of the *beings*. The subject created *alien presences* out of perceptually distorted noises by means of a belief program. The complex patterns of the noise coming through the spatially distorted and modified fields of the perceptual apparatus allowed creative construction of figures which satisfied current needs.

These distortions of the field are not static. The effects (maximal to the right) are seen as time-varying functions. Not only is there an apparent geometrical factor fixed to the body coordinates but there is a varying set of factors. It is the latter set that are locked in by an unconscious program for perception and for feelings. For the evocation of these programs in the LSD-25 state *the beliefs for the day* metaprogram determines the outcome. The patient says to himself *the presences seen come from outside me and my program storage*. These metaprogrammatic orders then are used in his computer to construct and modify whatever apparently comes in to create presences and at the same time to place the presences outside the computer itself. Thus these orders are essentially used twice: (1) For constructing a basic belief about the external reality of the presences and (2) for a display which demonstrates the results of computations using that belief. The belief is used on incoming signals with uncertain or distorted origins. Without LSD-25 this patient finds it difficult if not impossible to program such projections. He cannot use this basic belief counter to the powerful external reality program. It may be possible for him to use this belief without the LSD-25 state in possibly other extreme conditions, such as in the presence of white noise of large magnitude, the hypnogogic state, the dreaming state in sleep, or during hypnotic trance.

This patient says, "With the usual high levels of daylight in the summers or artificial light in the house, with the stimulation of me by other persons, with the usual high sound levels of e.r., all organized in demanding ways to call upon my purposes (integral to me), I cannot (or will not) program 'alien presences in the e.r.' Nor will I any longer so program 'presences' into other persons, as a consequence of my detection of the fact that I 'unconsciously programmed' presences of my own creation into other persons."

In most cases the unconscious programming is used to project one's own beliefs and "presences" into and onto other persons in the e.r. This is the easiest route to use and the hardest to detect. The detection is difficult because of (1) the resemblance of one human to another, (2) the apparently meaningless "noisy" signals other persons emit in every mode, and (3) the interlocking feedback relations between one's self and the important persons in the e.r. or the *apparent but effective* e.r. created by telephone, radio, television, motion pictures, books, etc.

Patients can thus have even evocable *proof* (false) of the *reality* (false) of their beliefs about another person. It is almost as if one can extend one's own brain-computer into that of another person by feedback and thus use the other as an actor, acting ("out there") the part assigned by one's own beliefs. Naturally, the performance is not perfect (see later **Interlock**).

If the roles are accepted by the other and acted upon as new programming, unconsciously, one cannot see these processes easily. If the other person asserts himself and opposes the assigned roles, one has an opportunity to examine these processes in one's self.

One can make the following self-assumptions about the above sources of information, in solitude, in the LSD-25 state: (1) inside one's own head; (2) from other beings, nonhuman; (3) from outer space intelligences; (4) from ESP with humans.

If one assumes a *transcendence* program, one's computer generates it according to one's own rules for *transcendence*. Programming can be assumed as if it came from self, or other humans, and/or from other beings. Modern scientists assume that under these conditions **information comes only** from self, i.e., from storage wholly within the human computer.

5

Note on the Potentially Lethal Aspects of
Certain Unconscious, Protohuman,
Survival Programs

It was found empirically that certain aspects of some programs carry the ability to destroy the individual biocomputer, or at least the ability to lead the way into potentially destructive action. A metaprogram to neutralize programs with self-destruction in them is necessary. The use of LSD-25 in self-analysis allows quick penetration to such buried lethality; a definite caution is advised in such use of this technique. Until such unconscious programs are found and thoroughly investigated, and understood in terms of the metaprogrammatic future, personal professional supervision (of a special type) is recommended. Such supervision should be over the whole period of investigation and (in detail) should be before, during, and after a session for at least several days. Some of the instinctual patterns of behavior stirred up in the process of the session apparently must be *acted-out* in order to be tested, understood and filed properly in the metaprograms for the future plans of the individual. In this phase, dangers to self arise.

The states of the *revelation* of the implanted deeper programs may involve the stages of childhood plus those presumed to have led Man (as an evolving primate) to civilization itself, and finally those leading into Man's own future beyond present accomplishments. Near the beginning (and sometimes later) of the LSD-25 analyses some survival programs (protohuman) may appear.

These programs include expressions of strong sexuality, gluttony, panic, anger, overwhelming guilt, sado-masochistic actions and phantasies, and superstitions. These are of amazing strength and power over the self-metaprogram. Much of this material is *wordless*: existing in the emotion-feeling-motivational storage parts of the computer, it usually has only poor representations in the *modeling*, clear thinking and verbal portions. The LSD-25 allows breakdown of the barriers between the emotional-wordless systems, and the wordfilled modeling systems by means of channeled uninhibited feeling and channeled uninhibited action. (This is one way that the *unconscious* is made *conscious* in a sometimes too rapid fashion.) If strong enough, the modeling systems (self-metaprogrammer) can receive the powerful currents of emotion in full force, *go along with them*, and eventually construct a vigorous operating model consonant with the desired ideal metaprograms but also with emotional power, built-in. If not strong enough, the self-metaprogrammer can be temporarily overwhelmed by the protohuman survival programs.

There is an additional caution in the use of these substances; the self-programmer must be strong enough to experience these phenomena and not make difficult-to-reverse mistakes in reprogramming or difficult-to-correct errors in new commitments in the external world. This is an area of human activity for the most experienced and strongest personalities, with the right training. **I do not recommend the use of these methods except under very controlled and studied conditions with as near ideal as possible physical and social environment and as near ideal as possible help from thoroughly trained empathic *matching* persons. The subject's short-term and long-term welfare must control all actions, all speech, and all transactions between each pair of persons present, unconsciously and consciously.**

¤ 6
Choice of Attending Persons During LSD-25 State
Used for Self-Analysis

The point is underscored: any action, facial appearance, word, sentence, tone of voice, or gesture on the part of the attending person can be used by the person in the LSD-25 state in the processes of penetration, elicitation, or reprogramming. Mistakes by the attending person here can have a devastating power and must be scrupulously avoided. Only mature, experienced, previously-exposed persons should be allowed in the e.r. during this critical time. The minimum possible number (1) of persons is best. This one person should, ideally, have been psychoanalyzed himself and have pursued his self-analysis with LSD-25 aid plus physical isolation and solitude. Short of this ideal, high-quality professional psychoanalytic training is a minimum ideal requirement, or careful selection of attending supervisors by such professionals. An exclusion test must be done on **any** potential attendant or therapist; he or she should have been personally through several LSD-25 sessions with the self-analysis metaprograms as the leading motivating instructions, and have penetrated to and beyond his own buried lethality and hostility. The professional selector should be thoroughly acquainted with such a potential aide, and evaluate the stages through which he or she has passed and achieved "permanently."

There can be special cases, less than the above ideal, but consonant with the principles enunciated. Some spouses or lovers (or both) have special understanding and interlocks which allow certain kinds of deep penetrations, elicitations and re-programmings, but not other kinds. If one of the pair has been through LSD-25 self-analysis training, it is possible (in special cases) to help the other member through a session or sessions as a standby monitor and positive love-object in the external reality. However, there should be some form of professional psychoanalytic control over such sessions. Such controls can vary from being implicit and in the nature of tactical and strategic advisory sessions to being e.r. supervisory, depending on the ego-strength and on the current stage of development of each member of the pair. Expert and informed clinical judgment after thorough clinical study is the best (known) instrument for such decisions.

7

Behavioral, Non-Isolation Replay of Protohuman
Programs: The Problem of Repetitive
Unconscious Replay

Certain kinds of programs in the human computer, usually below the ordinary levels of awareness, are circular. The circularity can be useful and needed, or misused (for example, in the maintenance of disparate and disturbing programs, L. Kubie 1939). A program in a certain patient says "Mother has abandoned baby, run to Daddy; Daddy beats me and leaves; Mommy comforts me and leaves; Daddy loves me and hurts me and leaves. Run to Mommy. Mommy has my sister, loves her, abandons me: run to Daddy; Daddy hurts. Daddy leaves. Run to Mommy. Mommy leaves. . .Mother has abandoned baby, etc." Again and again. When the patient was a baby this was the one important reality program; it became fixed, circular and carried into adulthood.

Such a program operates slowly or rapidly, and continuously. In the adult the real situation in the e.r. (external reality) cannot halt the circular program. Usually modeling in the reality is preeminent over such circularity. In this *circular case*, the e.r. is used to facilitate playback and maintain the strength of this *old model* program. Any important man or woman in the e.r. must, somehow, be made to fit into this "ancient model" program. An external observer sees a person with such a program repeating an unhappy pattern again and again over the years. The underlying perpetuated *baby* program is unavailable for inspection, replay and breaking of circularity by the owner as an adult.

At high doses LSD-25 reduces the relative strength of the e.r. program by enhancing the strength of other programs. (This occurs with 200 to 400 micrograms, and starts in the first hour and can continue for four or more hours.) LSD-25 can increase the strength of and activate basic models in storage; it also allows the self-metaprogramming orders (orders stored just before the LSD-25 maximum effect starts) to be carried out. Strong circular programs if present are likely to be replayed. The self-observer participates in the replay, but once again is programmed as relatively weak with respect to the replay program as he was as a baby or child at the time of the implanting episodes in the e.r. The external observer then sees a dramatic, repeat performance, again and again, of new replays.

Each replay is slightly different and gives the outside observer the feeling of a circular course not quite exactly repeating each time. The emotion expressed at first has all the desperate panic of the child; gradually the spectrum of intense emotion can be experienced and expressed progressively. With proper e.r., personnel, and responses from them, progress leads the circle gradually out of negative feelings into the regions of good feelings; the fear and other negative emotions are stripped off the circular program; good feelings are attached to replay; the self finally can see it operate with its new emotion and (possibly for the first time) examine its newly charged (positive) structure as it replays; reduce its importance on the unconscious priority list; and file it as a relic of childhood in the (inoperative or weakly operating) "history" file.

For a time, the self then feels free, cleaned out. The strength gained can be immense; the energy freed is double: the fight with the circular program is temporarily gone. Not only is the energy of self no longer absorbed in the fight but new program energy is available. For a short time, energy taken from the old circular program and the energy formerly expended in the fight may be available. So twice the energy of the circular program can be made available for use by the self-metaprogram in constructing new energy relations between desired programs directed toward ideals, aims, and goals. Adult love and sharing consonant with aspirations and reality (outside) gain strength and gain differentiation of response and of interlocks. Humor appears in abundance, good humor. Beauty is enhanced, the bodily appearance becomes youthful, with increased smiles and good-natured puns and jokings at a deep level of understanding and perspective. The babyish and the childish aspects of self are converted to adulthood with great strength of character, integrity, and loving. These positive effects can last as long as two to four weeks before re-assertion of the old program takes place.

FIGURE 1. SCHEMA OF THE LEVELS OF THE FUNCTIONAL ORGANIZATION OF THE HUMAN BIOCOMPUTER

LEVELS

XI	UNKNOWN	(above and in Biocomputer)
X	SUPRA-SPECIES-METAPROGRAMS	(beyond metaprogramming)
IX	SUPRA-SELF-METAPROGRAMS	(to be metaprogrammmed)
VIII	SELF-METAPROGRAM —— awareness	(to metaprogram)
VII	METAPROGRAMS METAPROGRAM STORAGE	(to program sets of programs)
VI	PROGRAMS PROGRAM STORAGE	(detailed instructions)
V	SUBROUTINES SUBROUTINE STORAGE	(details of instructions)
IV	BIOCHEMICAL ACTIVITY——NEURAL ACTIVITY——GLIAL ACTIVITY——VASCULAR ACTIVITY	(signs of activity)
III	BIOCHEMICAL BRAIN——NEURAL BRAIN——GLIAL BRAIN——VASCULAR BRAIN	(brain)
II	BIOCHEMICAL BODY——SENSORY BODY——MOTOR BODY——VASCULAR BODY	(body)
I	BIOCHEMICAL——CHEMICAL——PHYSICAL . . . . EXTERNAL REALITY	(external reality)

The boundaries between the body and the external reality are between Levels I and II; certain energies and materials pass this boundary in special places (heat, light, sound, food, secretions, feces). Boundaries between body and brain are between Levels II and III; special structures pass this boundary (blood vessels, nerve fibers, cerebro-spinal fluid). Levels IV through XI are in the brain circuitry and are the software of the Biocomputer. Levels above Level X are labeled "Unknown" for the following purposes: (1) to maintain future the openness of the system, (2) to motivate future scientific research, (3) to emphasize the necessity for unknown factors at all levels, (4) to point out the heuristic nature of this schema, (5) to emphasize unwillingness to subscribe to any dogmatic belief without testable reproducible data, and (6) to encourage creative courageous imaginative investigation of unknown influences on and in human realties, inner and outer.

Each part of each level has feedback-control relations with each part, indicated by the connecting lines. Each level has feedback-control with each other level. For the sake of schematic simplicity, many of these feedback connections are not shown. One example is an important connection between Levels VI through IX and X; some built-in, survival programs have a representative at the Supra-Self-metaprogram Level as follows:*"These programs are necessary for survival; do not attenuate or excite them to extreme values; such extremes lead to non-computed actions, penalties, illness, or death."* After construction, such a Metaprogram is transferred by the Self-metaprogram to the Supra-self-metaprograms and to the Supra-species-metaprograms for future control purposes.

(Note: See text and glossary for definitions of terms used.)

8

Basic Effects of LSD-25 on the Biocomputer:
Noise as the Basic Energy for
Projection Techniques

In the analysis of the effects of LSD-25 on the human mind, a reasonable hypothesis states that the effect of these substances on the human computer is to introduce *white noise* (in the sense of randomly varying energy containing no signals of itself) in specific systems in the computer. These systems and the partition of the noise among them vary with concentration of substance and with the substance used.

One can thus "explain" the apparent speed-up of subjective time; the enhancement of colors and detail in perceptions of the real world; the production of illusions; the freedom to make new programs; the appearance of visual projections onto mirror images of the real face and body; the projections and apparent depth in colored and in black-and-white photos; the projection of emotional expression onto other real persons; the synesthesia of music to visual projections; the feeling of "oneness with the universe"; apparent ESP effects; communications from "beings other than humans"; the lowered Cloze-analysis scores by outside scorers; the clinical judgment of the outside observer of *dissociation psychosis, depersonalization, hallucination,* and *delusion* in regard to the subject; the apparent increased muscular strength, and the dissolution and rebuilding of programs and metaprograms by self and by the outside therapist, etc.

The increase in *white noise* energy allows quick and random access to memory and lowers the threshold to unconscious memories (*expansion of consciousness*). In such noise one can project almost anything at almost any cognitive level in almost any allowable mode: one dramatic example is the conviction of some subjects of hearing-seeing-feeling God, when "way out." One projects one's expectations of God onto the white noise **as if the noise were signals**; one *hears the voice of God in the Noise*. With a bit of proper programming under the right conditions, with the right dose, at the right time, one can program almost anything into the noise within one's cognitive limits; the limits are only one's own conceptual limits, including limits set by one's repressed, inhibited, and forbidden areas of thought. The latter can be analyzed and freed up using the energy of the white noise in the service of the ego, i.e., a metaprogram *analyze yourself* can be part of the instructions to be carried out in the LSD-25 state.

The noise introduced brings a certain amount of disorder with it, even as white noise in the physical world brings randomness. However, the LSD-25 noise randomizes signals only in a limited way: not enough to destroy all order, only enough to superimpose a small creative "jiggling" on program materials and metaprograms and their signals. **This noisy component added to the usual signals in the circuits adds enough uncertainty to the meanings to make new interpretations more probable.** If the noise becomes too intense, one might expect it to wipe out information and lead to unconsciousness (at very high levels, death).

The major operative principle seems to be that **the human computer operates in such a way as to make signals out of noise and thus to create information out of random energies where there was no signal**; this is the "projection principle"; noise is creatively used in non-noise models. The information "created" from the noise can be shown by careful analysis to have been in the storage system of the computer, i.e., the operation of projection moves information out of storage into the perception apparatus so that it appears to originate in the chosen "outside" noisily excited system.

Demonstrations of this principle are multiferous: in a single mode, listening to a real acoustic physical white noise in profound isolation in solitude one can hear what one wants (or fears) to hear, human voices talking about one, or one's enemies discussing plans, etc. With LSD-25 one can use two modes: one can **listen** to white noise (including very low frequencies) and **see** desired (or feared) visions projected on the blank screen of one's closed eyes. One can, in profound isolation (water suspension, silence, darkness, isothermal skin, etc., in solitude) detect the *noise level of the mind itself* and use it for cognitional projections rather than sense-organ-data projections. Instead of **seeing** or **hearing** the projected data, one **feels** and **thinks** it. This is one basis of the mistake by certain persons of assuming that the projected thoughts come from outside one's own mind, i.e., *oneness with the universe*, the thoughts of *God in one*, extra-terrestrial beings sending thoughts into one, etc. Because of the lack of sensory stimuli, and lack of normal inputs into the computer (lack of energy in the reality program), the space in the computer usually used for the projection of data from the senses (and hence the external world) is available substitutively for the display of thinking and feeling.

As was stated by Von Foerster ("Bio-Logic," 1962):

> "The occurrence of such spontaneous errors is far from an uncommon event. Conservative estimates suggest about 10^{14} elementary operations per second in a single human brain. If we can believe the recent work of Hyden (1960) and Pauling (1961), these operations are performed on about 10^{21} molecules. From stability considerations (Von Foerster, 1948) we may estimate that per second from 10^{9} to 10^{11} molecules will spontaneously change their quantum state as a result of the tunnel effect. This suggests that from 10^{-3} to 10^{-1}% of all operations in the brain are afflicted with an intrinsic noise

figure which has to be taken care of in one way or another." And further (same reference):

. . ."The beginning of our century saw the fallacy of our progenitors in their trust in a fixed number of $\dot{m}$ propositions. This number constantly grows with new discoveries which add new variables to our system of knowledge. In this connection it may amuse you that in order just to keep the logical strength of our wisdom from slipping, the ratio of the rate of coalescing, $\dot{k}$, to the rate of discovery, $\dot{m}$, must okay the inequality

$$\frac{\dot{k}}{\dot{m}} > k \cdot \ln 2$$

I have the feeling that today, with our tremendous increase in experimental techniques, $\dot{m}$ is occasionally so large that the above inequality is not fulfilled, and we are left with more riddles than before.

"To this frustration to reach perfect truth we, children of the second half of the twentieth century, have added another doubt. This is the suspicion that noise may enter the most effective coalition, flipping an established 'false' into a deceptive 'true,' or, what might be even worse, flipping an irrelevant 'true' into an unwarranted 'false.'"

GROWTH HYPOTHESIS

1. One major biological effect of LSD-25 may be a selective effect on growth patterns in the CNS. Some parts of the CNS are thought to be specifically accelerated in their

local growth patterns, i.e., the systems which are selectively active during the LSD-25 state.

2. For these postulated growth effects there is an optimal concentration of the substance in the brain. With less concentration than the optimal there is merely an irritating stimulation of the CNS (below the levels of awareness). At the optimal concentration (in the non-tolerant state) the phenomena of the *LSD-25 state* occur. This is a phase of initiation of new growth in the CNS. [This phase is a state of mind analogous to that presumed to exist in the very young human (possibly beginning in the fetus or embryo).]

3. If additional material is administered, prolongation of this phase can be achieved within certain limits. With the maintenance of the optimal concentration of substance, this phase is prolonged (hours) until *tolerance* develops.

4. The phase of developed tolerance is thought to be (in addition to other things) the phase of the completion of the fast new growth. Most of the new biochemical and neurological connections are completed.

5. If continuous maintenance of optimal concentration for many hours (and ? days) after this initial phase is then achieved, growth may continue slowly.

6. The growth is not thought to be confined to the central nervous system. The autonomic nervous system may grow also.

7. If the optimal concentration is exceeded, the substance excites a "stress syndrome" (i.e., adrenal-vascular-G.I. tract, etc.). (This syndrome is separate from the *affective* results of the LSD-25 state which in certain individuals can cause a stress syndrome. I am not speaking of such individuals. I am speaking of more sophisticated observers who have been

through the necessary and sufficient experiences to be able avoid a stress syndrome in the LSD-25 state.)

8. At concentrations above the optimal there can be a reversal of the beneficial effects in the induced stress syndrome. Anti-growth factors are stimulated. Homeostasis is thus assured in the organism. A similar phenomenon can be seen with *negative* programming during the LSD-25 experience. **Reversal of growth may be programmed in by the self-programmer, unconscious metaprograms, or by the outside therapist or other persons.**

9. At concentrations above optimal the resulting stress syndrome is programmed into the autonomic nervous system and continues (beyond the time of the presence of the substance) to repeat itself until reprogrammed out days or weeks later.

10. At levels above optimal, the self-metaprogram loses energy and circuitry to autonomous programs; the ego disappears at very high levels.

This complex series of relations shows the delicate nature of the best state for remetaprogramming and of remetaprogramming itself. Until sophisticated handling (of these substances, the self-metaprogram, the person, the setting, the preparation, etc.) can be achieved, careful voluntary education of professional personnel should be done, and done carefully with insight. Selection of persons for training must be diplomatic and tactful; it is a strategy to be carried out cooperatively without publicity. Candor and honesty at deep levels is a prime requisite.

9

Summary of Basic Theory and Results for
Metaprogramming the Positive States
with LSD-25

1. LSD-25 facilitates the positive (reward, positive reinforcement) systems in the CNS. (Tables 4-8, 10 and Figs. 3-9)

2. LSD-25 inhibits the negative (punishment, negative reinforcement) systems in the CNS. (Tables 4-9 and Fig. 9)

3. LSD-25 adds *noise* at all levels, decreasing many thresholds in the CNS. (Table 2 and Fig. 9)

4. The apparent strengths of programs below the usual levels of awareness increase. (Figs. 3-5 and 9)

5. *Programmability* of metaprograms (*suggestibility*) increases, allowing more programming by the self-metaprogram and external sources [*hypersuggestibility* of H. Bernheim (1888), Clark Hull (1933).] (Fig. 9)

6. The continuous positive state (*positive reinforcement*, reward, pleasure) plus inhibited negative system activity causes increased positive reinforcement of the following:

    a. self
    b. one's own thinking
    c. thinking introduced by others
    d. other persons
    e. the given environment (r.r.)

  f. any given patterned complex input (i.e., music, paintings, photos, etc.). (Tables 9 and 10 and Fig. 9)

7. Subsequent to exposure, the effects fall off slowly over a two- to six-weeks period, during which period there is over-valuation of 6 (a-f). Residual effects can be detected up to one year.

8. Repeated exposures at weekly to biweekly periods for several months (years) maintain the above reinforcements if the above conditions, inputs and outputs can be reproduced. There is *reinforcement* of the positive reinforcements until the usual state before LSD-25 becomes negative.

◻ 10
Coalitions, Interlock and Responsibility

Von Foerster ("Bio-Logic," in *Biological Prototypes and Synthetic Systems*, Plenum Press, 1962) calls attention to the increasing survival times of increasingly large aggregates of connected matter which he defines as *coalitions*. Living systems are coalitions **par excellence**. A protozoan is a coalition of atoms and molecules forming membranes and sub-micro and micro structures which reproduce by collecting the same kinds of atoms and molecules from the environment to form new *identical* individuals. A sponge is a primitive coalition of protozoa with enhanced survival over any one protozoan. A man is a tightly organized coalition of cells, including some mobile *protozoa* (lymphocytes, macrophages, oligodendroglia, etc.). Von Foerster says that mammalian cells of **Homo sapiens** may be the most numerous cells on earth, i.e., these cells with their multiple level coalitions have the longest current survival time. (Table 2)

The nature of matter-matter coalitions and cell-cell coalitions and organism-organism coalitions are explored by Von Foerster. For a coalition to exist between any two entities, the dyad is connected by a bond or bonds which reduce the negentropy below the sum of the negentropy of each of the two entities separated (without a linkage). In this view the two entities when in coalition reduce the **physical information** available externally below the levels of that available from the two entities each unlinked and separated. The coalition as it exists thus appears to be something more than the mere sum of isolated parts.

84

However, the nature of the linkages in coalitions depends upon the level of aggregations discussed. In a man the coalitions include those between special atoms in spatial arrangements with others (alpha helices, etc.), special cells in spatial patterns (liver, brain, etc.), and *organism coalition tissues* such as circulatory, lymph, and autonomic nervous systems. The bones assure a maintenance of total form of the net coalition of a person under a *one g* gravitational field. The continuance of important aspects of the individual for inter-organism coalitions is based on shape maintenance despite g forces, radiation, heat, etc.

The rules within the coalitions at each level are different in that each level is somehow more than the sum of its separated individuals.

For coalitions to develop between individual humans, linkages of various sorts are developed: agreements are reached and thus the sources of new information from each member are reduced. To maintain a dyadic coalition, interlock between the two human computers is developed. Each human to human interlock is unique; but also each interlock is a function of other current and other past interlocks of each member and of learned traditional models.

Coalitions between humans are immense in number and have great complexity in their operations. Each adult individual has linkages extending to literally thousands of other individuals. The amount of time spent on maintenance of linkages is fantastic. The demands on one's self by the various coalitions uses up most of one's awake hours (and possibly most of one's sleeping hours).

To clarify the discussion we must carefully distinguish between an interhuman coalition operating here and now versus one whose past occurrences in the external reality are modeled in the human biocomputer. The here and now operations of the model of a past dyadic coalition can operate in the absence of a current instance of interhuman dyadic coalition or in its presence.

But the Model Operates Differently
in the Two Cases

With vigorous current e.r. interlock, the human biocomputer is busy with information exchange at all levels [verbal and non-verbal, digital and analogic, etc., (G. Bateson)]. The model projects expectations and predictions continuously as the interlock develops (as in McCulloch's model of the eye, 1961). The real inputs are compared with computed outputs in all modes.

The isolated solitudinous individual does not have a present coalition to work on, in, or with. He projects past coalitions and makes new models by making new coalitions, of the old ones. As such new relationships are established in his computer he settles logical discrepancies between old models and new ones, tends to abolish discontinuities of the logical consequences, his basic belief structures, and, if necessary, he changes the basic beliefs to have fewer discrepancies between the internal models.

Coalitions at all levels (from basic particles, atomic-molecular, to cellular-organismic, to human-human levels) have a polar, opposite, balancing set of forces, energies, drives, motivations. On the basic particle-atomic-molecular coalition level, this set can be called *electric charges*, with well-known coalitional rules (opposite attracts, like repels, quantal energy jumps, tunnelling effect, etc.). On the biological level of cells, the cell-cell coalitions have multiferous possibilities (such as meiosis, mitosis, fission, fusion, positive and negative tropisms, ingestion, excretion, etc.). As long as a cell has its own structure, it maintains only **structural relations** between molecules in itself: it is said (Duvigneau) that each and every atom in a cell is eventually exchanged for another new atom. The coalitions of a cell's atoms are temporary and in the mass last a most probable time characteristic of cell and atom types (lead in bone vs. sodium in brain, for example).

At this cellular level electric charges, on the average, establish gradients; the gradients vary with internal reality and external reality states; the atoms move in and move out, more or less rapidly depending on cell parts (nucleus, mitochondria, ribo-somes, etc.) and functional locus (intracellular fluids vs. genic structures, etc.).

An intra-organismic cell (in the mammals for example) has coalitions with other cells and with the organism. It has orders about its relations with neighbors, its origins, its meiotic or mitotic future (if any), its motility or sessility, its electrical activity, its chemical activity, where it stays or where it travels and on the average where and when it dies. Each cell is brought under the mass orders of all (of the organism) by carefully regulated rules of feedback and interconnections through chem-ical, physical and cellular means. The high-speed intercellular neuronal activity system penetrates most of the organism. The intercellular fluid flow penetrates everywhere and bridges the gap between the cell and the blood carriers. The blood system links the basic chemistry everywhere with transport (oxygen from outside, molecules from gut, hormones from pituitary, etc.). At the cellular level in the organism the coalitions are essential, the linkages myriad, and the cell is the well-fed and well-cared for *slave of the state* (the organism) and is killed if he breaks the orders for his type. Feedback is absolutely limiting here.

At the organism-organism level, the coalitions depend, some-what like the cellular level, on food, temperature, gravity, radi-ation, reproduction, one's own structure, individuals of other species of life, individuals of one's own species, communication intra- and inter-species, use of one's own computer (CNS plus), building and use of human artifacts (from tools to skyscrapers to rockets to non-living computers), and the control and the cre-ation of human relationships (money, credit, politics, science, books, periodicals, television, etc.).

A single human organism can have at least the following coalitions to deal with:

(a) **Parental**: till their death, and continuance as internal models.

(b) **Male-female**: continuously, at all ages, especially in the marriage coalition.

(c) **Financial**: individual (money) income and outgo is a multiple *general purpose* coalition sign. The amount of money whose flow is controlled by a given individual is, in general, a quantitative measure of coalition responsibility delegated to that individual by coalitions of many other individuals. An individual can be the controller of a coalition only with multiple consents, and hence control the flow of money into and out of that coalition.

(d) **Children**: exciting demanding coalitions develop with one's offspring. It is a challenge to renew and improve one's own coalition with each child as the child grows and expands his/her coalition powers.

(e) **Unconscious coalitions**: below the levels of awareness, one expects certain kinds of conditions in one's coalitions; some wishful thinking is expended in phantasied linkages. Contracts as written usually do not, cannot, incorporate explicit statements of unconscious commitments/desires. However, a contract can be misused in the service of wishful thinking — the courts see numerous cases of this kind.

The problems attendant upon breaking human-human coalitions can be smoothly worked out, be somewhat energetic, or can generate much heat, smoke and fire. The real bond energy left in the linkages usually can be dissipated at any rate desired; the fuss and furor (external energy dissipation) seems to be directly proportional to the energy in the bond and to the rate of bond dissolution, i.e., directly proportioned to the time taken and energy spent to obtain agreement on both sides of the human-human linkage. But the rate control and the necessities of agreement to break the coalition must be dispassionately and objectively evaluated. Unless one knows how to control the results, one desires to avoid exciting protohuman survival programs below the levels of awareness in either or both parties in the coalition; these programs require continuous care and maintenance.

Some essential factors of any and all human-human coalitions are circular feedback, distance rules, positive (attractive) and negative (repulsive) motives, excitation and inhibition rules and limits, and *coalition field* agreements. Each human coalition is formed in a *coalition field* surrounded by other coalitions with other individuals and with institutional agents. The connectivity of a given coalition with all other coalitions is multiple and complex. One is born and raised in a coalition field which is dynamic and growing; in this field the coalitions vary over a great range of apparent durations. Some coalitions are made to last beyond a single human lifetime; others to last a few minutes or hours or days or weeks.

The freed bond energy from a broken coalition is used to form new coalitions, or to strengthen others. For example, a resignation is preferable to a firing; a new pair of necessary coalitions can take the place of the old one with overlap and without break in services; or the duties of the old coalition are distributed over others.

The bond energies in human coalitions are of two types: attractive and repulsive; to maintain a viable coalition these links must be excited and inhibited by each member within certain limits of time, intensity, rate, etc. Sometimes a coalition has aspects of two persons pulling one another together with two ropes and, simultaneously, pushing one another apart with two poles; the coalition requires adjustment and readjustment of the two pushes and the two pulls involved. (The double-bind, G. Bateson)

Our concept of individual human responsibility rests on the above mappings of multi-level coalitions at each developmental age of the human being. Responsibility starts with a satisfactory coalition between one's self and the demanding 10^{12} cells of one's own body.

Responsibility continues with human-human coalitions, with interspecies coalitions (from immunity to bacteria, to eating plants and animals, to interspecies communication), with concepts of self (origins, maintenance, progress, destinations), and strong open communication of one's self with one's innermost realities.

In this paper the multiple levels of responsibility and the necessities for a strong autonomous character in order to pursue this research are underscored. In order to function effectively in human society the depths of the mind must be functioning relatively smoothly under the guidance of the self. To develop this degree of smooth function may require strong measures; these measures require strong educated handling.

⊓ 11
Participant Interlock, Coalitions with
Individuals of Another Species *

For approximately the last nine years the author has struggled with the problems of devising working models of the interspecies communication problem at a relatively high structured cognitive level. The major portion of the total problem has been found to be the author's own species, rather than the delphinic ones. There is apparently no currently available adequate theory of the human portion of the communication network, Man-Dolphin. The lack of such a theory has made it difficult for most scientists to see the reality of the problems posed in the interspecies program.

As long as the conscious-unconscious basic belief exists of the preeminence of the human brain and mind over all other earthside brains and minds, little credence can be obtained for the proposition that a problem of interspecies communication exists. Despite arguments based on the complexity and size of certain nonhuman mammalian brains, little if any general belief in the project has been instilled in the scientific community at large. Support has been obtained for further examination and demonstration of the large size, detailed excellence of structure, and description of the large dolphin brain; there is no lack of interest in this area. The faulting out comes in obtaining the operating

---

*Chapter 11 was published in part: Lilly, J. C. 1966. "Communication with Extraterrestrial Intelligence" (1965 IEEE Military Electronics Conf. Washington, D. C., Sept. 1965) IEEE Spectrum *3*: (3) 159-160.

91

interest of competent working scientists in evaluation of the performance of these large brains; interest and commitment of time and self are needed for progress.

The current effort on the part of this author is aimed at devising a program of encouragement for creating some models of the human end of the interspecies system which will illustrate, elucidate, and elaborate the basic assumptions needed to encourage interest and research effort in this area.

Each mammalian brain functions as a computer with properities, programs, and metaprograms partly to be defined and partly to be determined by observation. The human computer contains at least 13 billions of active elements, and hence is functionally and structurally larger than any artificially built computer of the present era. This human computer has the properties of modern artificial computers of large size plus additional ones not yet achieved in the non-biological machines. The human computer has "stored program" properties. "Stored metaprograms" are also present. Among the suggested properties are "self-programming" and "self-metaprogramming." Programming and metaprogramming language is different for each human depending upon developmental, experiential, genetic, educational, accidental, and self-chosen variables and elements and values. Basically the verbal forms for programming are those of the native language of the individual modulated by nonverbal language elements acquired in the same epochs of the development of that individual.

Each such computer has scales of self-measuration and self-evaluation. Constant and continuous computations are being done giving aim and goal-distance estimates of external reality performances and internal reality achievements. Comparison scales are set up between human biocomputers for performance measures of each and of several in concert. Each biocomputer models other biocomputers of importance to itself, beginning immediately post-partum, with greater or lesser degrees of error.

The phenomenon of "computer-interlock" facilitates mutual model construction and operation, each of the other. One bio-computer interlocks with one or more other biocomputers above and below the level of awareness any time the communicational distance is sufficiently small to bring the interlock functions above threshold levels.

In the complete physical absence of other external biocomputers within the critical interlock distance, the self-directed and other-directed programs can be clearly detected, analyzed, re-computed, re-programmed, and new metaprograms initiated by the solitudinous biocomputer itself. In the as-completely-as-possible-attenuated-physical-reality environment in solitude, a maximum intensity, a maximum complexity and a maximum speed of re-programming is achievable by the self.

In the field of scientific research such a computer can function in many different ways, from the pure austere thought processing of theory and mathematics, to the almost random data absorption of the naturalistic approach with newly found systems or to the coordinated interlocks with other human biocomputers of an engineering effort.

At least two extreme major kinds of methods of data collection and analysis exist for individual scientists: the artificially created, controlled-element, invented-devised-system methods; and the participant-observer interacting intimately experientially with naturally given elements with non-human (or human) biocomputers as interacting parts of the system. The first kind is the current basis of individual physical-chemical research, the latter kind is one basis for individual explorative first discovery research with large-brained (cf. human size) organisms. Sets of human motivational and procedural postulates for the interlock method of research with and on beings with biocomputers as large and larger than the human biocomputers are sought. Some of the methods sought are those of establishing long periods (months, years) of human-to-other organisms biocomputer interlock of a quality and value sufficiently high to merit interspecies communication efforts on both sides at an intense and dedicated, highly-structured level.

RETREATS FROM INTERLOCK

Some human scientists faced with non-human species who have brain-computers equal to or larger than their own, retreat from responsibilities of interlock research into a set of beliefs peculiar to manual, manipulating, bipedal, featherless, recording, dry, air-vocalizing, cooperating-intraspecies, lethal-predatory-dangerous, virtuous-self-image, powerful-immature, own-species-worshipping primates, with 1400 gram brains.

Specifically, human scientists faced with dolphins (with 1800 gram brains) retreat into several safe cognitive areas, out of contact with the dolphins themselves. The commonest evasion of contact is the assumption of a human **a priori** knowledge of what constitutes "scientific research on dolphins," i.e., a limited philosophical, species-specific, closed-concept system.

Common causes of retreat are too great fear of the dolphin's large size, of the sea, of going into water, of the Tropics, of cold water, etc. Another safe retreat is into the *let's see what happens if we do this* or the experimental "mucking around" region. Years can be spent on this area with no interlock achieved; successful evasion is thus continued endlessly.

Increasingly and frequently scientists are trying the *let's pretend we are non-existent (to the dolphins) observers and do a peeping-Tom-through-underwater-windows on them*, commonly called an "ethological approach." This activity also evades interlock research quite successfully.

Other cognitive traffic control devices to evade the responsibilities of close contact are appearing about as rapidly as each additional kind of scientist enters the arena with the dolphins:

icthyologists, zoologists, comparative psychologists, anthropologists, ethologists, astronomers each has had at least one representative of his field approach dolphins. Each one thinks up good and sufficient reasons for not continuing interlock research and not devoting his personal resources and those of his scientific field to such *far-out, non-applied, long-term, basic research.* Non-scientist-type persons also approach; most leave with similar sophistries. A few stay. Some who stay have an exploitative gleam in their eye: dollar-gleam, military-application-gleam, self-aggrandizement-gleam. Some persons stay because of a sense of wonder, awe, reverence, curiosity, and an intuitive feel of dolphins themselves.

The dolphin respecting (not *dolphin-loving*) persons (scientists or not) are the potential interlock group sought; dedication to dolphin-human interlock without evasions is a difficult new profession. The persons I know in this class are few, as of 1965. The few need help: facilities, assistance of the right sorts, privacy, few demands of other kinds, money, cognitive and intellectual back-up, encouragement, enlightened discussions, and, of course, dolphins. This is currently a necessarily lonely profession.

METAPROGRAMS FOR INTERSPECIES INTERLOCK

Several authors have proposed models of human and non-human communication based on purely logical, linguistic, and computer grounds. (See, for example, *Lincos*, a language for cosmic intercourse, by Freudenthal.) Such models suffer from one major defect: they lack the necessary experience in the proposer with interlock research with a non-human species; the storage banks of the theorizer are filled only with human-type interlock data. Of course this does not mean that these models are totally inapplicable, it merely assures a subtle pervasive anthropocentricity which may be inappropriate.

Among many possible theoretical approaches is one which I call the "participant theorist" approach. The theorist establishes an interlock with a non-human computer by whatever modes are possible, programs himself with open-ended hypotheses of a type thought to encourage him and to encourage the other computer, each to communicate. The resulting interactions between the two computers set up new programs, driven by meta-programs which say *establish communication with the other computer.* The new theory develops with the new data as each evolves in feedback with the other. Corrections are introduced in context almost automatically by reward-punishment interactions in response to errors on each side of the dyad.

OBSERVATIONS WITH TURSIOPS-HUMAN INTERLOCK:

MIMICRY AS EVIDENCE OF INTERLOCK

It has been found [with one non-human species (**Tursiops truncatus**) with a brain known to be sufficiently large to motivate the human end adequately] that a large daily commitment of hours to interlock is necessary for the human end, the order of 16 to 20 hours of the 24. The days per week must be at least five, and preferably six or seven. After 11 weeks of these hours, an approximate total of 1000 hours of interlock, the communication achieved via non-vocal and vocal channels was quite complex, and at the human end, the theories quite new and operationally successful, from an order-take-orders level to several higher levels.*

With dedicated interlock the conscious-unconscious reciprocal models of each computer in the other become workable within

---

*Lilly, J. C. 1967; Lilly, J. C., Alice M. Miller and Henry M. Truby, 1968. J. A. S. A. 43: 1412-1424.

the limits inherent in each participant. The limits set are also conscious-unconscious, at the human end, at least.

Such interlock participation and realistic model building and rebuilding avoid the sterile purity of the approach from the armchair. It assures interlock in most areas, including some interlock even in those areas forbidden to western "civilized man." The total necessities in each mode of expression are presented irrespective of taboos, inhibitions, bad theories, and blocks in either species. Areas to be loosened up are indicated unequivocally by each member of the dyad to the other by powerful methods. If communication attempts by one side are blocked in one area by the other, in many cases search tactics are employed until an open channel is found or until a channel is developed suitable to each end.

Early in the interlock, mutual rules are established regulating the muscle power and force to be used, and areas considered dangerous, the "absolutely" forbidden areas, the first channels to be considered, the limitations on the use of each channel, who is to have the initiative under what conditions, the contingencies surrounding feeding and eating, around sexual activities, arriving and leaving, sleeping, urination and defecation, the introduction of additional members of either species, and the use of props and evasions. The initial phase consumes most of this initial 1000 hours of interlock.

The consciousness-unconsciousness aspect of the initial period of interlock is an important consideration: if too much hostility-fear is present unconsciously the interlock becomes ritualistic and evasive. If the human end has too much unconscious energy involved in unconscious circuits of dependence on humans of the mother-child-father variety, fear-hostility may rupture the interlock suddenly. If powerful means of clearing out the unconscious excess-baggage circuits are used, one sees a sudden access to interlock of a depth and energy previously lacking in that human. A sudden willingness to participate at all levels effectively is generated and used as the computer is cleared of of unreasonable circular feedback programs below the level of awareness. This is at the human end of the system.

At the other-species end of the system, the selection of individuals for interlock is more hit or miss. We catch dolphins in the wild; we don't know how they select (if they do select) the group for us to catch. There seems to be some selection going on: most of the individuals we have worked with have none of our unconscious-hostility, unconscious-fear programs in their computers; at least not in the hands of our people in the Institute.* Rarely are very old ones caught.

It may be that dolphins in general cannot afford waste of the unconscious circuitry for such useless programs as hostility-fear-to-intelligent-other-individuals. The conditions for their survival in the wild require the utmost in fast and unequivocal cooperation and interlock with one another. The exigencies of air-breathing, of sharks, of storms, of bacterial diseases, of viral illnesses, of man's depredations, and of other factors require exuberance and whole-hearted participation (intraspecies) from each and every individual. Failure to interlock because of fear, hostility or other inner preoccupations leads to quick death and non-propagation of that type of computer.

Dolphins, correctly approached, seek interlock with those humans who are secure enough to openly seek them (at all levels) in the sea water.

With dolphins there are possible and probable interlock channels for humans. Anatomical differences limit the channels, as do human social taboos. Given a human with minimal inhibitions, the necessary sensitivity, skills in the water, courage, dedication, correct programming, and the necessary surrounds and support, there are many channels: sound-production-hearing; muscular-action-tactile-pressure-reception; presence-action-seeing; sexual

---

*Communication Research Institute, Miami, Florida and St. Thomas, U. S. Virgin Islands.

channels; feeding-eating; and such metachannel problems as initiative in use, cross-channel relations simultaneously with intrachannel control of signals, kinds of signals which can and cannot be decoded into information at each end, etc.

One channel we have disciplined ourselves and the dolphins to pursue is the air-borne vocal and hearing one.* In this channel we have found a clue to progress in the other channels: **if one is to be convincing in regard to showing a program and metaprogram *wish to communicate*, one mimics the other end's signals even though (temporarily) the signals make no sense, and one insists on having one's own signals mimicked on the same basis.** This leads to mimicry of our swimming patterns by the dolphins, for example, when we have mimicked theirs.

Mimicry seems to be one program for demonstrations of the present state of the model of the dolphin in us and of us in the dolphin. The adequacy of the functioning of the human in the man-dolphin interlock is measured by the feedback represented by mimicry. The mechanism is similar if not identical to that of a human child mimicking adult use of words (silently or vocally) not yet in the child's "storage" and "use" programs.

Plea for Further Research

In summary, a plea is made for the development of a theory of the communicator, human type, faced with a non-human communicator with a brain and presumed mind of a high quality. The theory should include open-ended, non-species-specific, general purpose, self-programming, mutual respect, voluntary dedication, participant theorist kinds of basic assumptions. Beyond these assumptions are those of the proper selection of participants, support, interest in the scientific community, and cooperation on an operating contributing level by open-minded professionals.

---

*OP. cit. J.A.S.A. 43: 1412-1424.

12
Summary of Logic Used in this Paper:
Truth, Falsity, Probability, Metaprograms
and Their Bounds

For the sake of clarity the following presentation of the logic employed in this paper is given.

It is quite apparent that there is at least a four-value logic employed. There are the usual 'true' and 'false' values; in addition there is another pair which in a shorthand way can be called 'as if true' and 'as if false.' Each of these four values can be applied to the external reality and to the internal reality of the human biocomputer.

The notation employed is as follows: for the external reality applications, 'true' and 'false' are rewritten without quotes. 'As if true' and 'as if false' are written with an asterisk ahead of the true and ahead of the false (*true, *false). For the internal realities situation, i.e., the occurrence of these values in the software of the human biocomputer, double quotation marks are placed around "true," "false," "as if true" and "as if false," ("*true" and "*false").

Externally checkable, observable reality, i.e., with external proof, uses the value system: true, false, *true and *false. In the internal reality, i.e., in the area of internal judgment, internal belief, in the self-metaprogrammer, the values are symbolized with quotation marks, "true" and "false" "*true" "*false."

In the internal reality case, for each of these values, there is a metaprogram which can be stated as follows: "define as true

100

(or false) a given metaprogram." (In the main body of the paper this is a basic belief for survival, for example.) A less intense metaprogram is "defined as if true a given metaprogram or defined as if false a given metaprogram." In the experiments on basic beliefs, "if defined as "true" then the metaprogram is "true" within limits to be determined," and "if defined "*true" then "true" within limits to be determined."

These various values may be modified with a judgment of their probability and with the defining of the desired intensity. The probability scale is 1.0 for absolutely certain, a gradation of probability down to the value 0 which is improbable and to -1 for impossible. Such values are applied to each of the four logic categories with regard to a specific metaprogram.

Such a logic system can be seen operating in the external human reality in coalitions of various sorts. A coalition can function 'as if an internal judgment' in the sense that it defines certain things as "true" which are then true within limits to be determined. The usual structure of human law seems to share this property. The concept of *consensus wisdom* (Galbraith) includes this logic system.

There are certain metaprograms and programs which have an imperative, externally-proven truth-falsity relationship which cannot be manipulated within the human biocomputer without danger to its existence. These metaprograms and programs can be considered as imperatives from some parts of the program level of the human biocomputer which must function as supra-self-metaprograms (i.e., there must be recognition of the "built-in," "necessary for survival nature" of these programs).

Some of these true programs are yet to be determined in biological science. The following have been determined: the necessity of obtaining food in response to hunger, the necessity of sexual activities and pleasure, adequate responses to pain and fear (such as freeze, flee, or fight).

Programs designed for survival of the body in a gravitational field take up a large fraction of the apparatus and of the time and energy of the human computer. The physiological limits of stimulation of the special senses must be closely maintained, i.e., not too high or too low levels of light, sound, and so forth. External temperatures and internal temperatures must be regulated within certain limits. Illnesses introduce new programs, including those illnesses which are the result of self-meta-programming.

Direct physical injury with physical trauma to the body have their own imperatives. The intake of certain gases into the respiratory system must be regulated very cautiously. Among these are oxygen, carbon dioxide, water vapor, carbon monoxide, nitrogen, xenon, krypton, nitrous oxide, and so forth. There are programs regulating the amount of liquid surrounding the body (for example, to avoid drowning), the amount of solids piled on top of the body (to avoid crushing), the total pressures of gases around the body (neither too much nor too little), the level of radiation, the level of elementary particles from outer space, or from artificial sources.

The various kinds of viruses, bacteria, fungi, algae, protozoa, and so forth, must be carefully regulated by proper programming.

Interactions of the human computer with other mammals and with supra-mammalian species must be programmed in an anticipatory way.

There must be regulation of information, the kind of information and the amounts from anywhere and from anyone for the best functioning of the human computer. There are such phenomena as "information-overload" and "information-deprivation." There are multiple programs for the regulation of the individual with respect to the society surrounding him, which have their own imperatives.

In summary, there are metaprograms which must be assumed

to be true in the sense of external reality and external proof. Each of these metaprograms has its own definition of that which is true or false. The 'as if true' and 'as if false' categories can only be applied to these metaprograms in temporary hypothetical consideration of their content but not in their performance in the real computer and in the real world. During the LSD-25 state certain of these programs must be considered as true (externally true and provable) in order to survive during the LSD-25 state. These matters are examined in more detail in other parts of this work.

13

Hardware, Software Relationships in the
Human Biocomputer *

Make the following simplifying assumptions in order to investigate some of the complex relationships between the metaprograms, programs and the neuronal activity in the central nervous system:

1. Assume an array of approximately 10^{10} neurons connected in the particular ways they are in the central nervous system.

2. Assume that the particular critical events in each neuron is the firing of an impulse into its axon.

3. Assume a method of control of this firing from outside the CNS.

4. Assume a method of pickup of the impulse discharged which can be transmitted to the outside of the CNS.

5. Assume that each impulse of each neuron in the 10^{10} array is recorded in a high-speed computer outside the CNS.

6. Storage of the time of occurrence of each impulse is stored as a separate datum.

---

*Levels IV-XI, Fig. 1.

7. Assume that for every second there are 10^{14} such impulses stored from the total CNS.

8. Assume that this external computer can, in a subsequent time period over 10^{10} channels, reproduce the time pattern of impulses stored, in the same time pattern in which they came into storage.

9. Test this hypothesis by a behavioral technique.

10. During a time in which the organism containing the bio-computer is doing some complex behavior such as speaking a sentence and writing a sentence at the same time, record completely the external behavior [color 3-D motion pictures, multiple channel tape (microphones, etc.)].

11. Store all of the neuronal signs of activity during the time of production of speech and of the writing.

12. In a subsequent time period, play back or call up from storage the patterns which were stored in the same sequence and put them out from the computer over 10^{10} channels into the CNS.

13. Record the subsequent behavior and compare this record with the previous external record of the behavior when the sentence was being produced.

14. The present theory states that behavior of the organism during the time of reproduction of the pattern will be very closely identical with the original occurrence of the behavior.

If the original hypothesis is correct, the two patterns of behavior as seen by camera, sound recorders, and so forth, will be identical. If something else is operating in the computer than control by neural impulses, the two behaviors will have differences, depending on the extent of the control. It may be that longer time patterns are needed in order to control all of the feedbacks (with, say, the endocrine and biochemical systems) which have longer time constants than the proposed experiment. There may have to be preconditioning periods which are also stored, before the two behavior sequences can be made identical.

With this model, we can ask many basic questions: for example, what is the physical set of events which gives rise to phenomena in the area of the phoneme, in the area of semantic levels of abstraction, in the areas of metaprogramming outside, and the use of language for programming?

With this technique, evaluation of drug effects on the central nervous system can have meaningful results in terms of the critical physical events taking place in the CNS. Analyses can be made of the kinds of programming and metaprogramming that take place in separate systems of the brain such as the neo-cortex, the meso-, paleo-, and archeo-cortices versus the sub-cortical systems such as the thalmus, the hypothalmus, mes-encephalon, etc. A systems analysis is then possible of the limbic system, the positively reinforcing and negatively reinforcing systems, the control of the pituitary, and the feedback control by the contents of the blood of the various parts of the CNS. Evaluation of the feedback relationships between all of these systems can then be specified in a quantitative way.

This formulation **objectifies the subjective** in a way in which experiments can be designed, not only to store the objective aspects of subjective events, but also to reproduce the subjective events from store. It permits quantitative analysis of the physical aspects of the subjective events outside of the CNS which originally created them.

It also permits of experiments in which a given CNS can control most (if not all) of the functions of a second CNS. The corresponding parts of the second CNS as compared to the first can be found and an evaluation made of the differences in thresholds, in area distributions of thresholds and in analogous areas between the two CNS's.

A more detailed proposal is given in the following Chapter 14.

Human Biocomputer: Biophysical Analysis and Control of
                     Brain
                     Activity-Program Levels (Figs. 2-9 &
                     Tables 3-10)

Program Level ⎞
              ⎬ relations
Brain Activity Level ⎠

(1.0)   Hypothesize a double connection to every CNS neuron
        of the 10^{10} array of neurons.
        a. The first connection picks up the firing sign (action
           potential) of each neuron.
        b. The second connection furnishes an electrical pulse
           (10^{-5} sec. duration) which fires each neuron, no
           matter its threshold for firing.
(2.0)   Hypothesize a method of storing signs of (1a) as they
        occur, in the storage of a huge computer, each sign
        stored by time and place of occurrence, over a time of
        1/2 hour (1800 sec., 1.8×10^9 micro sec.).
(2.1)   Record total behavior of organism over a time of 1/2
        hour.
(3.0)   At any time later, all stored signs are put out through
        connections (1b) in original sequence.
(3.1)   Record resulting behavior of organism for the 1/2 hr.
        of replay.

(4.0) *Questions:*

I. Does 3.1 record $\neq$, $\overset{\sim}{=}$, or $\equiv$ 2.1 record?

II. Does subjective life during 3.0 $\neq$, $\overset{\sim}{=}$, or $\equiv$ 2.0 interval? (See IX below.)

III. Is there memory of 2.0 during 3.0? Afterwards?

IV. Are 3.0 and 2.0 remembered as two time periods and event sequences?

V. Does psychophysical testing with objective records during 3.0 give identical results to same tests (using same time course) during 2.0? (Word test programmed on tapes with step distortions below the threshold for step detection, etc.)

VI. Other than (1a) need we store anything else? What about (a) membrane potential of each cell? (b) variations of M.P. over dendritic tree? (c) local concentrations of serotonin, nor-epinephrine, etc.? (d) previous history of firings for how long before chosen 1/2-hour period? (e) blood levels of critical substances? (f) glial activities and concentration of substances?

VII. Other than 1b need we control anything else? (See VI list of factors.)

VIII. Are 1a and 1b enough to specify and control, or does *molecular signal storage* introduce a measure of control independent of neuron firing?

IX. Does such detailed control of neuron firing give control of (a) program level and (b) metaprogram level, or is there another set of controlling variables and parameters?

X. Does this proposed system give control of (a) self-metaprogram and (b) supra-self-metaprogram levels? Does this system function as an absolute supra-self-metaprogram?

¤ 15
Metaprogramming the Body Image

Some of the most deeply entrenched and earliest acquired metaprograms are those of the personal body image of the human biocomputer. Among the programs of importance here are those of posture, walking stance, sitting patterns, lying down patterns and body posture during sleep. This metaprogramming interdigitates with that for acquired muscular skills of every sort, including writing, running, skiing, sports such as tennis, swimming, and so forth. These metaprograms also interdigitate with those of the use of the body during highly emotional states such as angry outbursts, sexual activities (both alone and with a partner), fright and flight patterns, and so forth.

The self-metaprogram feeds back on itself through the external body image seen in a mirror and through proprioceptive and postural feedbacks.

To investigate the proprioceptive and muscle tension aspects of the body image requires deep probing of programs combined with attempts to push every joint of the body beyond the limitations set by the current self-metaprogram. During such maneuvers to increase the range of motion at specific joints, one quickly discovers the joint capsules and muscles themselves have assumed anatomical limits which attenuate the range of possible motion at these joints. This is particularly true of the spinal joints and the pelvic joints (with the spine and with the femur). Similar considerations apply to the rib cage and the thoracic spine, the cirvical spine, as well as, the limb joints. By daily repeated regimes of reprogramming of the muscles and the joints, it is possible to begin to modify these entrenched programs.

During the primary state of LSD* it is possible to program in positive system activity during such exercises. Under these conditions the net effect of such stretchings and muscle exercises can be a positive system excitation and reinforcement of the new patterns. During the LSD state it has been noticed that the activities of the negative systems are attenuated and thus allow a greater range of muscle and joint stretching than without the LSD. It has also been noticed that it is possible to contract the desired muscles more fully in this state than during the usual state. Caution must be observed, however, because it is now possible to contract muscles to the point where muscles, joint capsules, ligaments, and tendons can be strained leaving residual, unpleasant local pains after the LSD primary state is ended.

During such exercises in the LSD state, it is possible to detect (by looking at the body image in a mirror during such exercises) the supra-self-metaprograms for the body image, both the positive and the negative ones. One can see the negative metaprogram, for example, as the projection of an aged and crippled body assumed to be too old to be capable of changing the body image. A positive projected metaprogram for example is that of an athletic young figure.

Certain kinds of negative attenuation and zeroing-out metaprograms are connected with pelvic movements. If there is a supra-self-metaprogram directed against the movements of sexual intercourse, these are reflected in body posture and in the range of use of the pelvis in other activities. Such metaprograms can be detected in the projected images (placed upon the mirror image of the body itself) by watching the posture of the pro-

_____

*Experiments with dextro-amphetamine in doses from 40-200 mgs show similar positively reinforcing pleasurable use of muscles, joints, posture-changes, etc., and inhibition of negatively reinforcing painful effects for several hours.

jected image and the range of programmable functional movements of the pelvis. The imagined dangers of sexual mating can be seen by the failure of this set of images to go through the full ranges of such motions. Reprogramming such anti-metaprograms requires the real body to go through the "forbidden" movements in order to investigate the anti-metaprograms. In general this requires more or less extreme exaggeration of the real body movements in order to break through the inhibitory aspects of the undesired metaprogram. Each individual will vary from others in the essential details, even as their metaprograms vary. A certain willingness to experience that which is feared most is absolutely essential as a basic metaprogram in order to achieve the new programming.

Cautions, once again, are in order here to avoid the narcissistic-self-worshipping-evasion of reprogramming in this area. The new areas of experience opened up can be rather seductive of themselves, because of the enhanced positive system activity during the LSD state. The necessity for regression and regrowth from times at which the natural developments were stopped can lead to further sticking of the metaprogramming at an earlier age on hedonistic grounds. Additional supra-self-metaprograms insisting on a natural evolution of the self-metaprogram towards a desired set of ideal metaprograms is necessary here to assure progress.

In older persons with well-developed characters these dangers are not as pressing as they are in younger subjects. However, the self-metaprograms involving the body image are also more entrenched in the older persons. More energy and dedication to the task at hand are needed in the older persons.

In those in whom obesity has become a problem, it is necessary to reduce the body weight to a more ideal level while these exercises in remetaprogramming of the body image are being carried out. In other words, it is necessary to carry out those real dietary and exercise instructions which lead to a real externally better body in the sense of physical health. Such a regime can reduce the probability of the onset of the typical diseases of old age, and with increasing health and activity, the remetaprogramming becomes more rewarding.

One metaprogram which has been worked out in great detail which may be of help to some persons is the set of exercises and dietary rules commonly called Yoga. These exercises assure new areas of stretching and new areas of breathing exercises which can enhance the physiologic functions of lungs and gut tract, as well as somatic musculature, joints, bones, and posture. In many ways these exercises assure adequate massage of the heart and blood vessels in such a way as to increase their activity along healthy lines. It may be that one can reduce the probability of a coronary attack, angina pectoris, and similar problems of the aged. Obviously other organs are also participating including liver, kidneys, spleen, and so forth.

In obesity the panniculus adiposus, the large fat store in the omentum and in the mesentery, severely limit functions of all of the viscera and limit the amount of stimulation that can be given these organs through such exercise. Such large fat reservoirs also require very large amounts of circulation of their own and hence require an increase in blood pressure to force that circulation.

Thus the external changes in the body image are reflected in internal changes throughout the body, in a self-reinforcing manner.

⌐ 16
Brain Models

TABLE 1

VIEWS OF ORGANISM: MODELS
1. Physical-chemical to quantum mechanical
2. Physiological (*structure and function*)
3. Modern psychological (*behavior*)
4. Classical psychological (*psyche*)
5. Evolutionary (*origins of life and species*)
6. Social, anthropological (*pre-historical, historical, current*)
7. Non-human intelligences
8. Religious, mystical (*supra-human entities*)

TABLE 2

VIEWS OF ORGANISM: MODELS
1. Physical-chemical: *series of millisecond to microsecond frozen* micro-pictures of patterns of neuronal activity, biochemical reserves, physical-chemical flows, energy-force-material exchange with outside sources-sinks; repeatability, reliability, signal/noise relations.

2. Physiological: partial integrated-over-time pictures of physical patterns: net results over seconds to days to years. Organism vs. environment generation of actions, signals.

3. Modern psychological: selection of certain aspects of

physical physiological data and models which show properties of modifiability, CNS model making, model comparison, storage, *learning, memory, physchophysical*.

4. Classical psychological: mental, subjective, *inside view*, psychoanalytic, solipsistic, ego-centered, personal models.

5. *Evolutionary*: gradual formation of basic physical-chemical units into organic particles, cells, organisms; formation of genetic codes and cytoplasmic orders; increasing sizes of cellular aggregations; formation of species; changes to new species; evolution of CNS; evolution of man from anthropoids; origins of speech.

6. Social, anthropological

7. Basic particles→aggregates→cells→tissues→organs→ organisms→ behavior

TABLE 3

KINDS OF "STIMULI"

1. Physical specifications: **endorgans**: kind and amount, timing, patterning of energy
2. Physiological specifications: **neuronal**: threshold values, patterns of neuron excitation (kind, place, impulses/ second)
3. Central nervous system specification: number of excited neurons, where, what impulse frequencies; buildup of central state in what systems, its kind.

TABLE 4

KINDS OF "RESPONSES"
1. Patterned musculo-skeletal:
    (A) **Starting** a feedback pattern with apparatus or with another organism
    (B) **Stopping** a feedback pattern
2. Patterned CNS-biochemical states generating musculo-skeletal responses:
    (A) Neutral
    (B) Net rewarding
    (C) Net punishing
    (D) Net ambivalent

FIGURE 2

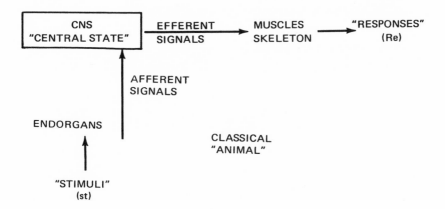

TABLE 5

KINDS OF CENTRAL STATES
  (0) Sleeping
  (1) Neutral
  (2) Activated
  (3) Inhibited
  (4) Rewarding
  (5) Punishing
  (6) *Disinhibited*
  (7) Integrative
  (8) Ambivalent

TABLE 6

PLACES IN CNS FOR "CENTRAL STATES"
  (0) Sleep system
  (1) Afferent projection systems
  (2) Efferent projection systems
  (3) Primary activation systems
  (4) Primary inhibition systems
  (5) Reward systems
  (6) Punishment systems
  (7) Integration systems
  (8) Pattern storage systems
  (9) Programming systems

TABLE 7

FEEDBACK "CAUSES" IN CENTRAL STATES
  1. Patterns of immediate results of outside *stimuli* (strength, place, timing).
  2. Patterns of immediate results of *responses.*
  3. Stored integrated *consequences* patterns.
  4. Continuous current cortical integration of selected past stored patterns and current results of outside *stimuli* and *responses.*

5. Cellular biochemical states of storage-depletion of specific substances in specific sites: reserves available in body.
6. Specific CNS biochemical states locally.
7. Built-in programs

TABLE 8

INTERLOCK: EXTERNAL REALITY PROGRAM
Systems
1. Afferent
2. Efferent
3. Reticular modulating $\pm$
4. Positive system phasing
5. Negative system phasing
6. Cortical storage and programming
7. Built-in programs

TABLE 9

NARCISSISTIC STATES through electrical stimulation of the brain, drugs, programming, and isolation: basic factors are:

1. Prolonged hyperactivie (+) systems.
2. Hypoactivity (−) systems.
3. Attenuation of external stimuli, responses, transactions.

TABLE 10

"CONVULSIONS" OF ORGASM-LIKE TYPE
If convulsion (behaviorally seen) includes prolonged hyperactivity of (+) systems, convulsions act as positive reinforcement with increased seeking and repetitions of ways of repeating the experience. (Dostoyevsky, Bickford, Sem-Jacobsen, Lilly).

FIGURE 3

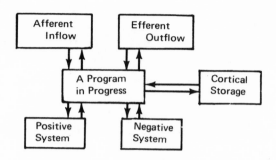

FIGURE 4

STORAGE

Data	*Place*
New, Current	Cortex
	Paleocortex
Older	Archeocortex
Inherited	Subcortex

FIGURE 5

SCHEMA OF PROGRAMS

Level	*Programs*	*Places*
1	New, Modifiable	Neocortex
	↓ ↑	↓↑ Paleocortex
2	Old, Fixed	Archeocortex
	↓ ↑	↓↑
3	Built-in	Subcortex

FIGURE 6

*A LARGE FRACTION OF THE BRAIN HAS
STIMULABLE ELEMENTS WHICH GIVE CONDITIONABLE
RESPONSES TO LOCAL ELECTRICAL STIMULATION
AT LOW LEVELS*

1. Neocortex-Projection systems (visual, acoustic, sensori-motor) — present, now
2. Paleo-Archeocortex-fixed, old patterns
3. Striate-mixed projection, positive-negative
4. Hypothalamus-septum and mesencephalon - positive and negative-present

FIGURE 7

*MOTIVATIONAL HIERARCHY OF CNS INSTRUCTIONS
(BRADY)*

Most (+)	Lat. Hypothalamus
	Ant. Med. Forebrain Bundle
	Orbitofrontal Cortex
	Amyagdala (cf. Powell et al.)
Least (+)	Entorhinal Cortex
Neutral (0)	Septal Area
Negative (−)	Fornix

FIGURE 8

Positive (+) & Negative (−) Systems:
Short vs. Long Train Effects

Positive	Negative
Neocortex-long	Neocortex-long
Hippocampus-long	
Amygdala-long	
	Amygdala-long
	Intralaminar Thal. N-short
Caudate N-short	
Lat. Hypothalamic N-short	Med. Hypothalamic N-short
Med. Forebrain Bundle-short	
Interpeduncular N-short	
	Central Gray-short

FIGURE 9

Primary State Induced by Hypnosis, LSD, Etc.

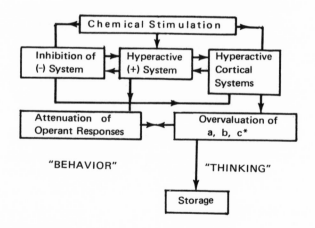

*a. Nearby Persons
 b. Current Thinking
 c. Emotional State

FIGURE 10

Second Train Durations

Single Zones in "Motor" Cortex

*(Noncortical).	Muscle response (to 1 pulse)
*"Move".	Muscle response (to train)
*"Stop".	Negative reinforcement threshold ("conditioned avoidance")
*"Start".	Positive reinforcement threshold ("self-stimulation")
*"Alerting".	Conditional stimulus ("detection")

FIGURE 11

(Short Trains)

Subcortical Nuclei "Positive" Zone

*"Stop".	(Spread to negative zone) muscle movements
*"Taming" - "Gentling".	Autonomic responses
*"Start".	Positive reinforcement "Self-stimulation"
*"Alerting".	Conditional stimulus threshold

FIGURE 12

(Ramp Schedule)

Single Zone in "Negative" Subcortical Nuclei

*"Escape" - "Anger".	Built-in somatic muscle patterns released
*"Fear".	Autonomic responses
*"Stop".	Negative reinforcement threshold ("conditioned avoidance")
*"Alerting".	Conditional stimulus threshold

Excerpts from "The Idiot" by Fyodor Dostoyevsky *

Examples of Extremely Active Positive-System State: Subjective Report, Special Type of Epileptic Seizure.

Dostoyevsky in a letter to Nikolai Strakhov.

> "For a few moments before the fit", he wrote to the critic Nikolai Strakhov, "I experience a feeling of happiness such as it is quite impossible to imagine in a normal state and which other people have no idea of. I feel entirely in harmony with myself and the whole world, and this feeling is so strong and so delightful that for a few seconds of such bliss one would gladly give up ten years of one's life, if not one's whole life."

Prince Leo Nikolayevich Myshkin:

> "He was thinking, incidentally, that there was a moment or two in his epileptic condition almost before the fit itself (if it occurred during his waking hours) when suddenly amid the sadness, spiritual darkness and depression, his brain seemed to catch

---

* pp. 8 and 258. Translated by David Magarshack. Penguin Books Ltd., Harmondsworth, Middlesex, England, 1960.

fire at brief moments, and with an extraordinary momentum his vital forces were strained to the utmost all at once. His sensation of being alive and his awareness increased tenfold at those moments which flashed by like lightning. His mind and heart were flooded by a dazzling light. All his agitation, all his doubts and worries, seemed composed in a twinkling, culminating in a great calm, full of serene and harmonious joy and hope, full of understanding and the knowledge of the final cause. But those moments, those flashes of intuition, were merely the presentiment of the last second (never more than a second) which preceded the actual fit. This second was, of course, unendurable. Reflecting about that moment afterwards, when he was well again, he often said to himself that all those gleams and flashes of the highest awareness and, hence, also of 'the highest mode of existence', were nothing but a disease, a departure from the normal condition, and, if so, it was not at all the highest mode of existence, but, on the contrary, must be considered to be the lowest. And yet he arrived at last at the paradoxical conclusion: 'What does it matter that it is an abnormal tension, if the result, if the moment of sensation, remembered and analyzed in a state of health, turns out to be harmony and beauty brought to their highest point of perfection, and gives a feeling, undivined and undreamt of till then, of completeness, proportion, reconciliation, and an ecstatic and prayerful fusion in the highest synthesis of life?' These vague expressions seemed to him very comprehensible, though rather weak. But that it really was 'beauty and prayer', that it really was 'the highest synthesis of life', he could not doubt, nor even admit the possibility of doubt. For it was not abnormal and fantastic visions he saw at that moment, as under the influence of hashish, opium, or spirits, which debased the reason and distorted the mind. He could reason sanely about it when the attack was over and he was well again. Those moments were merely an *intense* heightening of awareness — if this condition had to be expressed in one word — of awareness and at the same time of the most direct sensation of one's own existence to the most intense degree. If in that second — that is to say, at the last conscious moment before the fit — he had time to say to himself, consciously and clearly, 'Yes, I could give my whole life for this moment,' then this moment by itself was, of course, worth the whole of life. However, he did not insist on the dialectical part of his argument: stupor, spiritual darkness, idiocy stood before him as the plain consequence of those 'highest moments'. Seriously, of course, he would not have argued the point. There was, no doubt, some flaw in his argument — that is, in his appraisal of that minute — but the reality of the sensation somewhat troubled him all the same. What indeed was he to make of this reality? For the very thing had happened. He *had* had time to say to himself at the particular second that, for the infinite happiness he had felt in it, it might well be worth the whole of his life. 'At that moment,' he once told Rogozhin in Moscow during their meetings there, 'at that moment the extraordinary saying *that there shall be time no longer* becomes, somehow, comprehensible to me. I suppose,' he added, smiling, 'this is the very second in which there was not time enough for the water from

the pitcher of the epileptic Mahomet to spill, while
he had plenty of time in that very second to behold
all the dwellings of Allah."

⌑ Summary

Some general ideas from extrapolation and reworking of modern general purpose computer theory are used to explain and to control some of the subjective aspects of the operations of the human brain. An addition (for the peculiarly human brain) to the theory of the general-purpose computers is the concept of the *self-metaprogram* or the *internal programmer* present in the 10^{10} neurons assembly known as the human brain. The self-metaprograms operate between the huge storage and the huge external reality. Self-programming properties (in addition to stored program properties) are essential to understanding mental operations and resulting external general purpose behaviors such as speech and language. Stored programs and metaprograms are characteristic of the human.

The **self-organizing** aspects of computer programming and programs are now conceptually reasonable and realizable in modern non-biological computers. The human brain, a super-biocomputer, as it were, is a **parallel processor**—a realizable artificial machine with this structure has not yet been built. The actions of certain substances on the brain are explicable by this theory: examination of stored programs and re-programming are opened by LSD-25 (possibly by the introduction of small amounts of programmatic randomness, *noise*). In the child, automatic metaprogram implantation (or externally forced meta-programming), persisting as metaprograms below the levels of awareness in the adult, can be controlling for the later adult programs, adult thinking, and adult behavior. Energy can be taken from some of these automatic metaprograms and transferred to the self-metaprogram with special techniques and special central states, chemically evoked. Some automatic unperceived programs are essential to biological nurture, survival, etc. Examples of methods, of investigations and of results in self-analysis and self-metaprogramming are given.

⌑ Acknowledgements

The author is grateful for a National Institute of Mental Health Career Award (of the National Institute of Mental Health, N.I.H., Bethesda, Md. 1962-1967) which gave the time and impetus necessary for the conception and the writing of this work. The National Institute of Mental Health also furnished the wherewithal for some of the experiments during the term of the author's service (1953-1958) in the U. S. Public Health Service Commissioned Officers Corps, jointly at the National Institute of Mental Health and at the National Institute of Neurological Diseases and Blindness at the National Institutes of Health, Bethesda, Md. In addition, at various times, portions of the work were supported in part by grants from the Air Force Officer of Scientific Research, the National Science Foundation, the National Aeronautics and Space Agency, the National Institute of Neurological Diseases and Blindness, N.I.H., and G. Unger Vetlesen Foundation, and the Michael Tors Foundation. For this support the author expresses his gratitude.

The author wishes to express his appreciation to the Institute of the Philadelphia Association of Psychoanalysis and the Baltimore Institute for the opportunity to take his psychoanalytic research preparation and training analysis (1949-1956). In particular, he is indebted to Dr. Robert Waelder and the faculties of that period, including Drs. Gerald Pierson (dean), Henry Katz, George Sprague, Eli Marcowitz, Amanda Stoughton, Jenny Waelder-Hall, Anderson and Lewis Hill. Dr. Lawrence Kubie has been most helpful with his metatheoretical reformulations of psychoanalytic theory. Dr. Douglas Bond's insistance on the combined neurological and psychoanalytic training gave confidence when needed.

Over the years the necessity and inspiration for the pursuit of the logic and languages of artificial computers as related to the brain were learned from Warren McCulloch. An opportunity to pursue this area of research in depth was arranged by Dr. Walter Rosenblith in 1962. To the LINC group at Massachusetts Institute of Technology (now at Washington University, St. Louis) the author wishes to express appreciation for coursework, patient teaching and help with a LINC computer during its development phases — in particular Dr. Wesley Clark, Mary Allen Wilkes Clark, B. G. Farley, and Dr. Thomas T. Sandel contributed much needed time.

In many ways discussions of the materials of this work with Drs. Fred G. Worden, Charles Savage, Joel Elkes, Seymour Kety, Willis Harman, and Sidney Cohen have aided in its formulation, and have indicated the desirability of its publication.

I am grateful to my colleagues (past and present) in the Communication Research Institute for many invigorating discussions, including Gregory Bateson, Drs. Peter J. Morgane and Henry M. Truby.

◻ Glossary

1. **Communication:** the process of the exchange of information between two or more minds.

1a. **Communication:** the process of exchange of information between metaprogramming entities within two or more computers.

2. **Information:** the calculated mental results of the reception of signals from another mind and the computed composed context of the next reply to be formed into transmissible signals.

2a. **Information:** the data received, computed, and stored resulting from the reception of signals by a metaprogramming entity from another computer and the computed data in the ready state in the same entity for transmission to another computer through a similar set of signals.

3. **Mind:** the entity comprising all of the (at least potentially) self-detectable processes in a brain which are at such a level of program complexity as to be detected and at least potentially describable in programming language; the self-metaprograms within the brain.

3a. **Mind:** a form of metaprogram in the software set of a very large biocomputer which organizes metaprograms for the purposes of self-programming and of communication.

3b. **Mind:** the computer-brain-detectable portion of a supra-physical entity tied to the physical-biological apparatus:

the remainder of this entity is in the soul-spirit-God region and is detectable only under special conditions.

4. **Program:** a set of internally consistent instructions for the computation of signals, the formation of information, the storage of both, the preparation of messages, the logical processes to be used, the selection processes, and the storage addresses all occurring within a biocomputer, a brain.

5. **Metaprogram:** a set of instructions, descriptions, and means of control of sets of programs.

6. **Self-metaprogram:** a special metaprogram which involves the self-programming aspects of the computer, which creates new programs, revises old programs, and reorganizes programs and metaprograms. This entity works only directly on the metaprograms, not the programs themselves; metaprograms work on each program and the detailed instructions therein. Alternative names are *set of self-metaprograms,* "self-metaprogramming entity," or the *self-metaprogrammer.*

MAJOR METAPROGRAMS

1. External Reality Metaprogram

This metaprogram operates programs with interlock with the outside-body-systems. These systems include all of external reality; human beings are a defined part of the external reality.

This metaprogram seems to be absent only in special states and even then possibly is only **relatively attenuated**, not completely absent. The states in which it is attenuated include sleep, coma, trance, anaesthesia, etc.

The above states cause centrally conditioned reductions of the stimulation arriving from the external reality. It is also possible to attenuate the external reality stimuli themselves.

In the profound physical isolation, external reality excitation of the CNS is attenuated to minimum possible levels in all modes. If in profound physical isolation, one adds a metaprogrammatically active substance to the brain (such as LSD-25), further attenuation of the external reality stimuli can be achieved and the *ego* (self-metaprogram) is more fully activated. If in profound physical isolation one adds sleep, trance, or anaesthesia (light levels), these give external reality cut-off and cessation of e.r. (external reality) excitation of the central nervous system (and of the "mind").

The external reality metaprogram is increased in its intensity in high excitation states; interlock with the external reality can be increased by these means.

2. Self-metaprograms

These metaprograms include all of those entities which are usually defined as *ego, consciousness, self,* and so forth.

The interlock of the self-metaprograms with the external reality metaprograms can be attenuated by special techniques including sleep, LSD-25 plus isolation, anaesthesia, etc.

The apparent strength of these metaprograms can be enhanced in certain cased by LSD-25 plus dextro-amphetamine, psychic energizers, etc.

3. Storage Metaprograms

These metaprograms have two aspects: there is the active storage process in which the inputs from e.r. and from self are connected to storage: there is the active output process in which the self is connected directly to storage. To achieve these connections there are the *search* metaprograms. The nature of these programs varies depending upon special conditions. It varies in *free association* states, hypnogogic states, dreaming states, etc. LSD-25 and similar agents allow a special state in which the self-metaprograms can directly consciously explore much of the storage itself. In this particular state the self-metaprograms and the search-metaprograms operate coextensively in such a way as to reveal the innermost files of the storage directly to self.

4. Autonomic (Nervous System) Programs

The autonomic nervous system has built-in properties which are definitely programmatic rather than metaprogrammatic. The relationships between these and the self-metaprogram are second order. These autonomic programs do not exist directly in self-metaprograms. These programs include the programs for the gastro-intestinal tract, for sex, for anger, for fright, etc. These programs can be modified by the self-metaprogram; once started their detailed carrying-out is automatic.

5. Body Maintenance Programs

These are programs which cut across the lines of the previous ones and include such conscious-unconscious programs as the needs and the carrying out of sleep, exercise, correct food, environmental temperature regulations, clothing, etc. The realities of the **body maintenance** in the external reality are included in these programs.

6. Family-Love-Reproduction-Children Program

This is also an aspect of the external reality metaprogram and here is separated out as one of the basic programs within that one.

Depending upon the individual computer there can be many more programs; some may be devised as above, others cut across the above boundaries. Such divisions, in the last analysis, are artificial and reflect the tendency of a human to think and act disintegrated into categories rather than as an integrated smoothly operating holistic computer.

7. Survival Metaprograms

Survival Priorities are used in case of threat to structural and/or functional integrity of the entities named: the order is that of relative importance in the sense that the one below in the list will be sacrificed, abandoned, penalized, or changed in order to save, maintain, integrate, or educate the one above in the series.

A threat is defined as internal (mental) information (which when above threshold) anticipates and predicts immediate or delayed destruction, mutilation, confinement, abandonment, damnation, ostracism, solution (lysis) of continuity, compromised integrity, moral encroachment, severe ethical insult, voluntary seduction, unconscious entrancement, slavery, etc.

In non-threatening educative processes the listing is more flexible: any entity may, for a time, be placed at the head of the new list. This survival priorities list may remain intact in this order in the depths below awareness. It is evoked in states of fatigue which begin to generate information above the threat threshold.

O.   The Soul-spirit: this concept includes life after mortal death, reincarnation, the immortal entity, that which is God-given, none of which is in current Science. This is currently considered by some persons as the most valuable of all the available entities. Depending on the needs of the definer, this entity may be educable, may have higher ethical strivings than current ones, may store information of certain kinds, may develop skills in certain areas, may carry these capabilities within it to the next state after the current mortal physical reality is left, etc.

1.   Ego-mind Entity: one's mind and mental self are valued above the body (and in those with the above religious belief, below the soul).

2.   Body: it is obvious that one values one's body less than one's mental self; however, at times one can be forced to act as if the list did not have this order but the opposite. Sometimes the mind shuts down, leaving the body to its survival battle alone.

3.   Lover: starting with the prototypic father and mother models and moving to wife or husband models.

4.   Child: one's own child.   5. Siblings.   6. Parents.

7.   Valued friends.   8. Humans in general.

KEY TO CATEGORIES IN REFERENCES AND BIBLIOGRAPHY

B   study of certain literature in biology

C   computers

H   hypnosis

I   psychiatry

L   logic

M   brain and mind models

N   neuropsychopharmacology

O   psychology

P   psychoanalysis

T   communication

◻ References

(See also the Categorized Bibliography, page 145)

Category	Page	
M*	3 60	Ashby, W. Ross. 1952. *Design for Brain.* John Wiley. New York. 260 p.
M	3	———— . 1962. "What is Mind? Objective and Subjective Aspects in Cybernetics." Chapter in *Theories of the Mind.* Jordan M. Scher (ed.). The Free Press of Greece, New York and Macmillan: New York, London. pp. 305-313.
O	3	Bartlett, Sir Fredric. 1858. *Thinking.* "An Experimental and Social Study." Basic Books, Inc., Publishers, New York. 203 p.
I & M	3 84	Bateson, Gregory, Don D. Jackson, Jay Haley, and John Weakland. 1956. "Toward a Theory of Schizophrenia." Behavioral Sci. I: 251-264.
H	3 9 75	Bernheim, H. 1888. *Hypnosis and Suggestion in Psychotherapy.* "A Treatise on the Nature and Uses of Hypnotism." Translated from the 2nd revised ed. by C. A. Herter. 1964.University Books, New Hyde Park, N. Y. 428 p.
L	3	Birkhoff, Garrett and Saunders MacLane. 1948. *A Survey of Modern Algebra.* The Macmillan Co., New York. 450 p.
B	3 91	Blakeman, J., Alice Lee and Karl Pearson. 1902. "A Study of the Biometric Constants of English Brain — Weights and Their Relationships to External Physical Measurement." Biometrica 4: 408-467.
N	3 41	Blum, Richard and Associates. 1964. *Utopiates.* "The Use and Users of LSD-25." Atherton Press, New York. 303 p.
L	xvii 3	Bourbaki, Nicholas. (pseud.) 1957. Scientific American. May. p.88.
N	3	Bradley, P. B., C. Elkes and J. Elkes. 1953. "On Some Effects of Lysergic Acid Diethylamide (LSD-25) in Normal Volunteers." J. Physiol. (London). *121*: 50 p.

---

* See key to categories, page 135.

Category	Page	
N	3	Bradley, P. B. and J. Elkes. 1953. "The Effect of Amphetamine and D-Lysergic Acid Diethylamide (LSD-25) on the Electrical Activity of the Brain of the Conscious Cat." J. Physiol. (London) *120:* 13 p.
M	119	Brady, Joseph V. 1960. "Temporal and Emotional Effects Related to Intracranial Electrical Self-Stimulation." Chapter 3 in *Electrical Studies of the Unanesthetized Brain.* Estelle R. Ramey and Desmond S. O'Doherty, Ed. pp. 52-77.
O	3	Bruner, Jerome S., Jacqueline J. Goodnow and George A. Austin. 1956. *A Study of Thinking.* John Wiley & Sons, Inc., New York; Chapman & Hall, Ltd., London. 330 p.
L	xx 3	Carnap, Rudolf. 1942. *Introduction to Semantics.* Harvard Univ. Press, Cambridge, Mass. 256 p.
L	xx	————. 1943. *Formalization of Logic.* Harvard University Press, Cambridge, Mass. 159 p.
L	xx 3	————. 1945. "Foundations of Logic and Mathematics." Vol. 1 No. 3 Int'l. Encyclopedia of Unified Science. Vols. I & II: Foundations of the Unity of Science. Univ. of Chicago Press, Chicago, Ill.
L	xx	————. 1947. *Meaning and Necessity. A Study in Semantics and Modal Logic.* Univ. of Chicago Press, Chicaco, Ill. 210 p.
T	3	Cherry, Colin. 1957. *On Human Communication. A Review, A Survey, and A Criticism.* The Technology Press of M.I.T. and John Wiley & Sons, Inc., New York: Chapman & Hall, Ltd., London. 333 p.
L	3	Churchman, C. West, Russell L. Ackoff and E. Leonard Arnoff. 1957. *Introduction to Operations Research.* John Wiley & Sons, Inc., New York, London. 645 p.
H	3	Clark, John Howard (U.K.) 1967. "The Structure of Hypnotic Procedure." 5th International Congress on Cybernetics. 11-15 Sept. 1967. Namur, Bruxelles, Belgium.
M	117	Clements, Betty G., John W. Bossard and Reginald G. Bickford. 1957. "Auras of Pain and Pleasure (sound motion picture of recording of seizures in two patients.)" EEG and Clin. Neurophysiol. *9.* Abst. 12:571.

Category	Page	
N	3	Cohen, Sidney. 1965. *The Beyond Within.* "The LSD Story." Atheneum, New York. 268 p.
M	3	Colby, Kenneth Mark. 1955. *Energy and Structure in Psychoanalysis.* The Ronald Press Co., New York. 154 p.
B	3	Dobzansky, Theororius. 1955. *Evolution, Genetics and Man.* John Wiley & Sons, Inc., New York; Chapman & Hall, Ltd., London. 398 p.
P	3 117	Dostoyevsky, Fyodor. 1960. *The Idiot.* Translated by D. Magarshack. Penguin Books Ltd., Harmondsworth, Middlesex, England.
B	119	Duvigneau. See Standard Biochemistry Text.
N	3	Elkes, Joel J. 1961. "Psychotropic Drugs. Observations on Current Views and Future Problems" in Lectures on Experimental Psychiatry. Univ. Pittsburgh Press. pp. 65-114.
I	3	Elkes, Joel. 1963. "Subjective and Objective Observation in Psychiatry." The Harvey Lectures. Ser. 57. Academic Press. pp. 63-92.
N	3	Elkes, C., J. Elkes, and W. Mayer-Gross. 1955. "Hallucinogenic Drugs." Lancet 268: 719.
N	3	Elkes, Joel. 1957. "Effects of Psychosomimetic Drugs in Animals and Man." Chapter in *Neuropharmacology.* H. A. Abramson (ed.). New York. pp. 205-95.
B, N	3	Elkes, J. 1958. "Drug Effects in Relation to Receptor Specificity Within the Brain: Some Evidence and Provisional Formulation" in *Neurological Basis of Behavior.* Ciba Foundation Symposium. Little, Brown & Col, Boston. pp. 302-336.
B, N	3	———— . 1960. "Drugs Influencing Affect and Behavior: Possible Neural Correlates in Relation to Mode of Action." Chapter V in *The Physiology of Emotions.* A. Simon, C. C. Herbert and R. Strause (eds.). Charles C. Thomas, Publisher, Springfield, Ill. pp. 95-150.
C	3	Feigenbaum, Edward A. and Julian Feldman (eds.). 1963. *Computers and Thought.* McGraw-Hill Book Co., Inc., New York, San Francisco, Toronto, London. 535 p.
O	3	Freud, Sigmund. 1966. The Standard Edition of the Complete Psychological Works of Sigmund Freud.

Category	Page	
		James Strachey, Anna Freud (eds.). Vols. *I-XXII* (1881-1936). London, Hogarth Press and the Institute of Psychoanalysis.
N	3	Freud, Sigmund. 1885. "Uber die Allgemeinurikung des cocains" (on general effect of cocain). (Lect. 5 Mar. 1885) Med. Chirug. Centrabbl. 1885 7 Aug. *20*: 374-376 & comm. Abs. Auth. Inhals wiss arb. 10.
N	3	————— . 1885. "Beitrag zur Kenntniss der cocaïnwirkung" (a contribution to the knowledge of cocaine). Wiener Med. Wochen. *35* (5): cols. 129-133 Abs. Auth. Inhals wiss arb. 10.
N	3	————— . 1887. Bemerkung uber cocaïnaucht und cocaïnfurcht mit Beziehung auf einen Vortag W. W. Hammonds (comments on cocaine addiction and cocaine fear with ref. to a lecture by W. W. H.) Wiener Med. Wochen. *37* (28): cols. 929-932 Abs. Auth. Inhals arb. 17.
N	3	————— . 1885. "Gutactan uber das Parke cocaïn (report on Parke's cocaine) in Gutt Uber die verschiedenen cocaïn-Praparati und deren Wirkung" (on cocaine & effects). Wiener Med. Wochen. *26* (32): 1036.
L, C	3 94	Freudenthal, Hans. 1960. *LINCOS, Design of a Language for Cosmic Intercourse*. L.E.J. Brouwer, E.W. Beth, A. Heyting (eds.). North-Holland Publishing Co., Amsterdam. 224 p.
T	3 98	Galbraith, J. K. 1958. *The Affluent Society*. Houghton, Mifflin, Boston.
H	3 18	Gill, Merton M. and Margaret Brenman. 1961. Hypnosis and Related States. Psychoanalytic Studies in Regression. International Universities Press, Inc., New York. 405 p.
B	3	*Handbook of Physiology*. 1959. Section 1: *Neurophysiology* Vol. I. John Field, H. W. Magoun and Victor E. Hall (eds.). Am. Physiol. Soc. Waverly Press, Inc., Baltimore, Md. 1-779 pp.
B	3	*Handbook of Physiology*. 1960. Section 1: *Neurophysiology*. Vol. II. John Field, H. W. Magoun and Victor E. Hall (eds.). Am. Physiol. Soc. Waverly Press, Inc. Baltimore, Md. 781-1440 pp.

140

Category	Page	
B	3	*Handbook of Physiology*. 1960. Section 1: *Neurophysiology*. Vol. III. John Field, H. W. Magoun and Victor E. Hall (eds.). Am. Physiol. Soc. Waverly Press, Inc. Baltimore, Md. 1441-1966 pp.
B	3	*Handbook of Physiology*. 1964. Section 4: *Adaptation to the Environment*. D. B. Dill, E. F. Adolph and C. G. Wilber (eds.). Am. Physiol. Soc. Waverly Press, Inc., Baltimore, Md. 1056 p.
B, M	3	"Homeostatic Mechanisms." 1958. Report of Symposium June 12-14, 1957. Brookhaven Symposia in Biology No. 10: 1-209 BNL 474 (C-25). Office Technical Services, Dept. Commerce, Washington, D. C. 270 p.
L	xx *3*	Hilbert, David and W. Ackerman. 1950. *Principles of Mathematical Logic*. Robert E. Luce (ed.). Chelsea Publishing Co., New York. 172 p.
O	3	Hilgard, Ernest R. 1956. *Theories of Learning*. Appleton-Century-Crofts, Inc., New York. 563 p.
H	3 9 75	Hull, Clark L. 1933. *Hypnosis and Suggestibility*. "An Experimental Approach." The Century Psychology Series. R. M. Elliott (ed.). D. Appleton-Century Co., Inc., New York, London. 416 p.
M	3	"Human Decisions in Complex Systems." 1961. Conference Chairman and Conference Editor Warren W. McCulloch. Ann. N. Y. Acad. Sci. *89*: 715-896.
L, O	3 49	Huxley, Aldous. 1952. *Heaven and Hell*. Harper & Brothers, New York. 103 p.
L, O	3 49	————. 1954. *Doors to Perception*. Harper & Bros., New York
M	3 80	Hyden, H. 1960. "The Neuron" in *The Cell*. Vol. *4*: 1. Academic Press, New York. 305 p.
O, N, T. M	3 9	James, William. 1929. *The Varieties of Religious Experience*: "A Study in Human Nature." Longmans, Green & Co., New York, London, Bombay and Calcutta. 526 p.
O	3 9	————. 1950. *The Principles of Psychology*. Vols. I & II. Dover Publications, Inc., New York.
M, B	3	Jeffress, Lloyd A. (ed.). 1951. *Cerebral Mechanisms in Behavior*. The Hixon Symposium. John Wiley & Sons, Inc., New York: Chapman & Hall, Ltd., London. 311 p.
P	3	Kubie, Lawrence. 1939. "A Critical Analysis of the

Category	Page	
		Concept of a Repetition Compulsion." Int. J. Psa. *20*: 390-402.
P	3	Kubie, Lawrence. 1950. *Practical and Theoretical Aspects of Psychoanalysis*. International Universities Press, Inc., New York. 252 p.
H	3	Lasker, Eric G. 1967. "Computerized Induction of Hypnosis." 5th International Congress on Cybernetics. 11-15 Sept. 1967. Namur, Bruxelles, Belgium.
N, O	3	Leary, Timothy and Richard Alpert. 1963. "The Politics of Consciousness-Expansion. The Harvard Review *I*: 43-54 p.
N	3	Leary, Timothy, George Litwin, and Ralph Metzner
	34	(eds.). 1963. "The Subjective After-effects of Psychedelic Experiences: A Summary of Four Recent Studies." The Psychedelic Review *I*: 18-26.
N	3	Leary, Timothy, Ralph Metzner, and Richard Alpert.
	35	1964. *The Psychedelic Experience: A Manual Based on the Tibetan Book of the Dead*. University Books, New Hyde Park, N. Y.
B, M	86	Lettvin, J. Y., H. R. Maturana, W. S. McCulloch, and W. H. Pitts. 1959. "What the Frog's Eye Tells the Frog's Brain." Proc. I.R.E. *47* (11): 1940-1959.
O, L	3	Lewin, Kurt. 1936. *Principles of Topological Psychology*. McGraw-Hill Book Co., Inc., New York and London. 231 p.
P	3	Lewin, Bertram. 1950. *The Psychoanalysis of Elation*.
	21	W. W. Norton, New York.
L	3	Lewis, Clarence Irving and Cooper, Harold Langford. 1932. *Symbolic Logic*. The Century Philosophy Series, S. P. Lambrecht (ed.). The Century Co., New York and London. 506 p.
T, P	xxii	Lilly, John C. 1956. "Mental Effects of Reduction of
	4	Ordinary Levels of Physical Stimuli on Intact,
	17	Healthy Persons." In Psychiat. Res. Report *5*.
	60	American Psychiatric Assn., Washington, D. C. pp. 1-28.
	13	———— . 1957. "Stop and Start Systems" in *Neuropharmacology*. Transactions of the Fourth Conference, Josiah Macy, Jr. Foundation. Princeton, N. J. pp. 153-179.

142

Category	Page	
	13	Lilly, John C. 1958. "Some Considerations Regarding Basic Mechanisms of Positive and Negative Types of Motivations." Am. J. Psychiat. *115*: 498-504.
	13	—————. 1958. "Rewarding and Punishing Systems in the Brain" in *The Central Nervous System and Behavior*. Transactions of the First Conference, Josiah Macy, Jr. Foundation. Princeton, N. J. p. 247.
	13	—————. 1959. "Stop and Start Effects" in *The Central Nervous System and Behavior*. Transactions of the Second Conference, Josiah Macy, Jr. Foundation and National Science Foundation. Princeton, N. J. pp. 56-112.
T, P	3 29 59	Lilly, John C. and J. T. Shurley. 1961. "Experiments in Solitude, in Maximum Achievable Physical Isolation with Water Suspension, of Intact Healthy Persons." Symposium, USAF Aerospace Medical Center, San Antonio, Texas, 1960. In *Psychophysiological Aspects of Space Flight*. Columbia Univ. Press, New York. pp. 38-247.
B, T	3 93	Lilly, John C. 1963. "Critical Brain Size and Language." Perspectives in Biol. & Med. *6*: 246-255.
O, M, T	64	—————. 1967. *Mind of the Dolphin: A Nonhuman Intelligence*. Doubleday & Company, Garden City, N. Y. 331 p.
M, L	3 102	McCulloch, Warren S. 1965. *Embodiments of Mind*. The M.I.T. Press, Cambridge, Mass. 402 p.
T, L	3	Miller, George A. 1951. *Language and Communication*. McGraw-Hill Book Co., Inc., New York. 298 p.
C, T	3	Muses, C. A. (ed.). 1962. *Aspects of the Theory of Artificial Intelligence*. Proc. 1st Int'l. Symp. On Biosimulation, Locarno. 1960. Plenum Press, New York. 283 p.
M, C	3	Pask, Gordon. 1962. "The Simulation of Learning and Decision-Making Behavior." Chapter VIII in *Aspects of the Theory of Artificial Intelligence*. C. A. Muses (ed.). The Proc. 1st Int'l. Symp. On Biosimulation, Locarno. 1960. Plenum Press, New York. pp. 165-210.
M	3 15	—————. 1964. "A Discussion of Artificial Intelligence and Self-Organization" in *Advances in Computers*. Franz. L. Alt and Morris Rubinoff. Vol. 5. Academic Press, New York, London. pp. 109-226.

Category	Page	
M	3 14	Pask, Gordon. 1966. "A Cybernetic Model for Some Types of Learning." Bionics Symposium 3-5 May, 1966. Dayton, Ohio. WADD Tech. Rept.
B	3 80	Pauling, Linus. 1961. "A Molecular Theory of General Anesthesia." Science *134*: 15-22.
O	3 14	Pavlov, I. P. 1957. *Experimental Psychology and Other Essays.* Philosophical Library, New York.
O	3	Piaget, Jean. 1956. *The Origins of Intelligence in Children.* Translated by Margaret Cook. International Universities Press, Inc., New York. 419 p.
L, T	3	Polya, G. 1954. *Patterns of Plausible Inference.* Vol. *II* of *Mathematics and Plausible Reasoning.* Princeton Univ. Press, Princeton, New Jersey. 190 p.
M	119	Powell, Ervin W., Jane Haggart, Elsie Goodfellow and William T. Niemer. 1957. "Hypothalamic Seizures from Stimulation of Rhinencephalon and an Isocortex in Cat." Neurol. 7: 689-696.
P, O	3	Rappaport, David. 1951. *Organization and Pathology of Thought.* Selected Sources. Translation and commentary by D. Rappaport. Columbia Univ. Press, New York. 785 p.
B	3	Rensch, Bernard. 1960. *Evolution Above the Species Level.* Columbia Univ. Press, Morningside Heights, New York. 419 p.
T	3	Rioch, David Mck. and Edwin A. Weinstein (eds.). *Disorders of Communication.* Proc. Assoc. for Res. in Ner. and Mental Dis. Dec. 7-8, 1962. New York, New York. Vol. *XLII.* The Williams & Wilkins Co., Baltimore. 519 p.
M	3	Rosenblith, Walter A. (Ed.). 1961. *Sensory Communication.* Symposium on Principles of Sensory Communication. (Endicott House 1959). M.I.T. Press and John Wiley & Sons, Inc., New York. 844 p.
B	xxv *3*	Schrodinger, Erwin. 1945. *What is Life? The Physical Aspects of the Living Cell.* Univ. Press, Cambridge, England: Macmillan, New York.
M	117	Sem-Jacobsen, C. W. 1968. "Depth-Electrographic Stimulation of the Human Brain and Behavior." Charles C Thomas, Springfield, Illinois. 200 p.
O	3 15	Skinner, B. F. 1957. *Verbal Behavior.* Appleton, New York.
O	xxviii *3*	Snow, C. P. 1959. *The Two Cultures and the Scientific Revolution.* Cambridge Univ. Press, New York. 58 p.

144

Category	Page	
L	xx 3	Tarski, Alfred. 1946. *Introduction to Logic and to the Methodology of Deductive Sciences.* Oxford Univ. Press, New York.
M, L	3 81	Von Foerster, Heinz. 1948. *Das Gedächtnis.* Deuticke, Vienna. 21 p.
M, L	3 79 84	———— . 1962. "Bio-Logic" in *Biological Prototypes and Synthetic Systems.* Eugene E. Bernard and Morley R. Kare (eds.). Vol. *I*, Plenum Press, New York. pp. 1-19.
M, L, B	3	Von Foerster, Heinz and George W. Zopf, Jr. (eds.). 1962. *Principles of Self-Organization.* Transactions of Univ. Ill. Symposium on Self-Organization, Robert Allerton Park, June 8-9, 1961. International Tracts in Computer Science and Technology and their Applications. Vol. *9*. A Pergamon Press Book. The Macmillan Co., New York. 541 p.
L, T	xxii 3	Von Neumann, John and Oskar Morgenstern. 1944. *The Theory of Games and Economic Behavior.* Princeton Univ. Press, Princeton, N. J. 625 p.
C, M	3	Von Neumann, John. 1958. *The Computer and the Brain.* Yale Univ. Press, New Haven, Conn.
P	3	Waelder, Robert. 1960. *Basic Theory of Psychoanalysis.* International Univ. Press, New York. 273 p.
C	3	Wegener, Peter (ed.). 1964. *Introduction to System Programming.* Proceedings of a symposium held at the London School of Economics 1962. Academic Press, London and New York. 316 p.
L	xx 3	Whitehead, Alfred North and Bertrand Russell. 1925-1927. *Principia Mathematica.* 3 Vols. 2nd ed. Cambridge University Press, Cambridge, Mass.
T	3	Whorf, Benjamin Lee. 1959. *Language, Thought and Reality.* Selected Writings. John B. Carroll (ed.). Technology Press, M.I.T. and John Wiley & Sons, Inc., New York and London. 278 p.
M	3	Wooldridge, Dean E. 1963. *The Machinery of the Brain.* McGraw-Hill Book Co., Inc., New York, San Francisco, Toronto, London. 252 p.

Categorized
*Bibliography**   *B, M**

Adrian, Edgar D.   1947. *The Physical Background of Perception.*
                         Clarendon Press, Oxford, England.
Ashby, W. R.   1945. "The Physical Origin of Adaptation by Trial
                         and Error." J. Gen. Psych. *32*: 13-25.
Ashby, W. Ross   1952. *Design for a Brain.* John Wiley & Sons, Inc.,
                         New York.
Ashby, W. Ross   1962. "The Self-Reproducing System" in *Aspects
                         of the Theory of Artificial Intelligence.* C. A.
                         Muses (ed.). (Proc. 1st. Int'l. Symp. on Bio-
                         simulation. Locarno, 1960). Plenum Press, New
                         York. pp. 9-18.
Ashby, W. Ross   1962. "What is Mind? Objective and Subjective
                         Aspects in Cybernetics." Chapter in *Theories of
                         the Mind.* J. M. Scher (ed.). The Free Press of
                         Greece, New York and Macmillan: New York,
                         London. 305-313 pp.
Bonin, Gerhardt Von   1950. *Essay on the Cerebral Cortex.* C. C. Thomas,
                         Springfield, Ill.
Brady, Joseph V.   1960. "Temporal and Emotional Effects Related to
                         Intracranial Electrical Self-Stimulation." Chapter
                         3 in *Electrical Studies of the Unanesthetized
                         Brain.* Estelle R. Ramey and Desmond S.
                         O'Doherty, Ed. pp. 52-77.
Chance, Britton,   1964. "Cyclic and Oscillatory Responses of Meta-
A. Ghosh   bolic Pathways Involving Chemical Feedback
J. J. Higgins   and Their Computer Representations." Ann.
P. J. Maitra   N. Y. Acad. Sci. *115* (2): 1010-1024.
Clements, Betty G.,   1957. "Auras of Pain and Pleasure (sound motion
John W. Bossard and   picture of recording of seizures in two patients)".
Reginal G. Bickford   EEG and Clin. Neurophysiol. *9.* Abst. 12:571.
Eccles, G. C.   1953. *The Neurophysiological Basis of Mind.* Clar-
                         endon Press, Oxford. 191 p.
Evans, C. R.   1964. "Dreaming: an Analogy from Computers."
E. A. Newman   New Scientist *24*: 577-579.
Fair, Charles M.   1963. *The Physical Foundations of the Psyche.*
                         Wesleyan University Press, Middletown, Conn.
Freud, Sigmund   1953. *On Aphasia, a Critical Study.* Int'l. Univ.
                         Press, New York.

---

*See key to categories, page 135.

146

Categorized
Bibliography   **B, M**

Head, Sir Henry   1963. *Aphasia and Kindred Disorders of Speech.*
                       Vols. *I* and *II.* Hafner Publishing Co., New York.

Hess, Walter R.   1954. *Diencephalon, Automatic and Extrapyram-*
                       idal Functions. Grune & Stratton, New York.

Jackson, J. Hughlings 1958. *Selected Writings.* James Taylor (ed.). Basic
                       Books, New York.

Kappers, C. U. Ariens 1960. *The Comparative Anatomy of the Nervous*
G. Carl Huber   *System of Vertebrates, Including Man.* Vols. I,
Elizabeth Caroline   II, III. Hafner Publishing Co., New York.
   Crosby

Lettvin, J. Y.   1959. "What the Frog's Eye Tells the Frog's Brain."
H. R. Maturana   Proc. I.R.E. *47* (11): 1940-1959.
W. S. McCulloch
W. H Pitts

MacKay, Donald M.   1962. "Theoretical Models of Space Perception" in
                       Aspects of the Theory of Artificial Intelligence.
                       C. A. Muses (ed.). (Proc. 1st Int'l. Symp. on
                       Biosimulation. Locarno 1960) Plenum Press,
                       New York. pp. 83-102.

McCulloch, Warren S.   1943. "A Logical Calculus of the Ideas Imminent
W. Pitts   in Nervous Activity." Bull. Math. Biophys. *5*:
                       115-133.

McCulloch, Warren S.   1945. "A Heterarchy of Values Determined by the
                       Topology of Nervous Nets." Bull. Math. Bio-
                       phys. *7*: 89-93.

———————   1952. *Finality and Form.* American Lectures Series
                       No. 11. C. C. Thomas, Springfield, Illinois. 63 p.

———————   1965. *Embodiments of Mind.* The M.I.T. Press,
                       Cambridge, Mass. p. 402.

Newman, E. A.   1965. "Human Dream Processes as Analogous to
C. R. Evans   Computer Programme Clearance." Nat. (Lon-
                       don) *206* (4983): 534.

Pask, Gordon   1962. "The Simulation of Learning and Decision-
                       Making Behavior" in *Aspects of the Theory of*
                       Artificial Intelligence. C. A. Muses (ed.). (Proc.
                       1st Int'l. Symposium on Biosimulation, Locarno
                       1960.) Plenum Press, New York. pp. 165-210.

———————   1964. "A Discussion of Artificial Intelligence and
                       Self-Organization" in *Advances in Computers.*
                       Franz L. Alt and Morris Rubinoff (eds.). Vol. *5*
                       Academic Press, New York, London. pp. 109-
                       226.

Categorized Bibliography	**B, M**
Pask, Gordon	1966. "A Cybernetic Model for Some Types of Learning." Bionics Symposium 3-5, 1966. Dayton, Ohio. WADD Tech. Rept.
Penfield, Wilder Theodore Rasmussen	1950. *The Cerebral Cortex of Man; A Clinical Study of Localization of Function.* Macmillan, New York. 248 p.
Penfield, Wilder Lamar Roberts	1959. *Speech and Brain-Mechanisms.* Princeton University Press, Princeton, N. J. 286 p.
Pitts, Walter Warren S. McCulloch	1947. "How We Know Universals: The Perception of Auditory and Visual Forms." Bull. of Math. Biophys. *9*: 127-147.
Powell, Ervin W., Jane Haggart, Elsie Goodfellow, William T. Niemer	1957. "Hypothalamic Seizures from Stimulation of Rhinencephalon and an Isocortex in Cat." Neurol. 7: 689-696.
Ramey, Estell R. Desmond S. O'Doherty (eds.)	1960. *Electrical Studies on the Unanesthetized Brain.* P. B. Hoeber, Inc., New York. 423 p.
Rensch, Bernard	1960. *Evolution Above the Species Level.* Columbia University Press, New York. 419 p.
Rosenblith, Walter A. (ed.)	1961. *Sensory Communication.* Symposium on Principles of Sensory Communication. (Endicott House, 1959). M.I.T. Press and Wiley & Sons, Inc., New York. 844 p.
Scher, Jordon M. (ed.)	1962. *Theories of the Mind.* Free Press of Glencoe, New York. 748 p.
Schmitt, Francis O. (ed.)	1962. *Macromolecular Specificity and Biological Memory.* The M.I.T. Press, Cambridge, Mass. 119 p.
Schrödinger, Erwin	1945. *What is Life? The Physical Aspect of the Living Cell.* Univ. Press, Cambridge, England; Macmillan, New York. 91 p.
Scheer, Daniel E. (ed.)	1961. *Electrical Stimulation of the Brain: An Interdisciplinary Survey of Neurobehavioral Integrative Systems.* Univ. of Texas Press (for the Hogg Foundation for Mental Health). Austin, Texas.
Sem-Jacobsen, C. W.	1968. "Depth-Electrographic Stimulation of the Human Brain and Behavior." Charles C. Thomas, Springfield, Illlnois. 200 p.
Sherrington, Sir Charles Scott	1920. *The Integrative Action of the Nervous System.* Yale Univ. Press, New Haven, Conn.

148

Categorized
Bibliography

B, M

Von Foerster, Heinz

1962. "Bio-Logic" in *Biological Prototypes and Synthetic Systems.* Eugene E. Bernard and Morley R. Kare (eds.). Vol. I. Plenum Press, New York. pp. 1-12.

————

1962. "Circuitry of Clues to Platonic Ideation" in *Aspects of the Theory of Artificial Intelligence.* C. A. Muses (ed.). (Proc. 1st Int'l. Symp. on Biosimulation. Locarno 1960). Plenum Press, New York. pp. 43-81.

Von Neumann, John

1958. *The Computer and the Brain.* Yale Univ. Press, New Haven, Conn. 82 p.

L

Birkhoff, Garrett
Saunders MacLane

1948. *A Survey of Modern Algebra.* Macmillan. New York. 472 p.

Boole, George

1948. *The Mathematical Analysis of Logic; Being an Essay Towards a Calculus of Deductive Reasoning.* Philosophical Library. New York. 82 p.

Carnap, Rudolf

1942. *Introduction to Semantics.* Harvard Univ. Press. Cambridge, Mass. 256 p.

————

1943. *Formalization of Logic.* Harvard Univ. Press, Cambridge, Mass. 159 p.

————

1945. *Foundations of Logic and Mathematics.* Vol. I., No. 3, Int'l. Encycl. of Unified Science, Vols. I & II: Foundations of the Unity of Science. Univ. of Chicago Press, Chicago, Ill.

————

1947. *Meaning and Necessity, A Study in Semantics and Modal Logic.* Univ. of Chicago Press, Chicago, Ill. 210 p.

Culbertson, James T.

1958. *Mathematics and Logic for Digital Devices.* Van Nostrand. Princeton, New Jersey. 224 p.

Hilbert, David
W. Ackerman

1950. *Principles of Mathematical Logic.* Robert E. Luce (ed.). Chelsea Publishing. New York. 172 p.

Lewis, Clarence Irving
Cooper H. Langford

1932. *Symbolic Logic.* The Century Co. New York and London.

Nyquist, Harry
Harry S. Black

1933. *Theory of Feedback Systems.* U. S. Patent No. 1,894,322. Milburn, New Jersey.

Shannon, C. E.

1949. *The Mathematical Theory of Communication*, p. 21. Univ. Ill. Press, Urbana, Ill.

————
W. Weaver

1964. *The Mathematical Theory of Communication.* Univ. of Ill. Press, Urbana, Ill. 125 p.

Categorized
Bibliography

Tarski, Alfred	**L**
	1946. *Introduction to Logic and to the Method-ology of Deductive Sciences.* 2nd Ed. Revised & translated by Olaf Helmer. Oxford Univ. Press, New York. 239 p.
Von Neuman, John Oskar Morgenstern	*Theory of Games and Economic Behavior.* Princeton Univ. Press. Princeton, New Jersey. 625 p.
Whitehead, Alfred North Bertrand Russell	*Principia Mathematica.* 2nd Ed. 3 Vol. 1925-27. Vol. 1, to 1956. Cambridge Univ. Press. Cambridge , Mass.
Wiener, Norbert	1948. *Cybernetics; or Control and Communication in the Animal and the Machine.* Wiley & Sons. New York. 194 p.

	N
Abramson, H. E. (ed.)	1954. *Conference on Neuropharmacology.* Transactions. Josiah Macy, Jr. Foundation. New York.
Bradley, P, B. J. Elkes	1953. "The Effect of Amphetamine and D-lysergic Acid Diethylamide (LSD-25) on the Electrical Activity of the Brain of the Conscious Cat." J. Physiol. *120:* 13. London.
Bradley, P. B. C. Elkes J. Elkes	1953. "On Some Effects of Lysergic Acid Diethylamide (LSD-25) in Normal Volunteers." J. Physiol. (London). *121:* 50.
Eccles, J. C.	1953. *The Neurophysiological Basis of Mind.* Clarendon Press. Oxford, England.
Eiduson, Samuel Edward Geller Arthur Yuwiller Bernice Eiduson	1964. *Biochemistry and Behavior.* Van Nostrand, Princeton, New Jersey. 554 p.
Elkes, C. J. Elkes W. Mayer-Gross	1955. "Hallucinogenic Drugs." Lancet *268:* 719.
Evarts, Edward V. W. Landau et al.	1955. "Some Effects of Lysergic Acid Diethylamid and Bufotenine on Electrical Activity in the Cat's Visual System." Am. J. Physiol. *182:* 594-598 pp.
Evarts, Edward V.	1956. "Brain Effects of LSD in Animals" in *Lysergic Acid Diethylamide and Mescaline in Experimental Psychiatry.* Grune & Stratton, New York, London. p.55
————	1956. "Some Effects of Bufotenine and Lysergic Acid Diethylamide on the Monkey." Arch. Neurol. & Psychiat. *75:* 49.

Categorized
Bibliography

N

Kety, Seymour S.

1960. "A Biologist Examines the Mind and Behavior." Science *132*: 1861-1870.

Killam, Eva K.
H. Gangloff
B. Konigsmark
K. F. Killam

1959. "The Action of Pharmacologic Agents on Evoked Cortical Activity." In *Biological Psychiatry*. J. H. Masserman (ed.). Grune & Stratton New York.

Killam, K. J.
E. K. Killam

1958. "Drug Action on Pathways Involving the Reticular Formation" in *Reticular Formation of the Brain*. H. H. Jasper et al. (eds.). Little, Brown, Boston, Mass. p.111.

Konorski, Jerzy

1948. *Conditioned Reflexes and Neuron Organization*. Univ. Press. Cambridge, England. 267 p.

Magoun, Horace

1958. *The Waking Brain*. C. C. Thomas, Publisher Springfield, Illinois. 138 p.

Marrazzi, A. S.
E. R. Hart

1955. "The Possible Role of Inhibition at Adrenergic Synapses in the Mechanism of Hallucinogenic and Related Drug Actions." J. Nerv. & Ment. Dis. *122*: 453.

Uhr, Leonard Merrick
James G. Miller
(Eds.).

1960. *Drugs and Behavior*. Wiley & Sons. New York. 676 p.

Unger, Sanford M.

1963. "Mescaline, LSD, Psilocybin and Personality Change, a Review." Psychiat. *26*: 111-125.

T

Cherry, Colin

1957. *On Human Communication: A Review, A Survey, and A Criticism*. Cambridge Technology Press of M.I.T. Cambridge, Mass. 333 p.

Chomsky, Noam

1957. *Syntactic Structures*. Mouton. 's-Gravenhage. 116 p.

Freudenthal, Hans

1960. *Lincos, Design of a Language for Cosmic Intercourse*. North-Holland Publishing Co., Amsterdam.

MacKay, Donald M.

1956. "Towards an Information-Flow Model of Human Behavior." Brit. J. of Psychol. *XLVII* (1): 30-43.

Miller, George A.

1951. *Language and Communication*. McGraw-Hill. New York. 298 p.

Morris, Charles W.

1945. *Foundations of the Theory of Signs*. Vol. I, No. 2, Int'l. Encycl. of Unified Science, Vols.

Categorized
Bibliography

T

I & II: Foundations of the Unity of Science, Univ. of Chicago Press. Chicago, Ill.

Pierce, John R. — 1961. *Symbols, Signals and Noise: The Nature and Process of Communication.* Harper. New York.

Poincaré, Henri — 1952. *Science and Hypothesis.* Dover Publications. New York. 244 p.

Whorf, Benjamin L. — 1956. *Language, Thought and Reality: Selected Writings.* Cambridge Technology Press of M.I.T., Cambridge, Mass. 278 p.

Wiener, Norbert — 1948. *Cybernetics: or Control and Communication in the Animal and the Machine.* Wiley & Sons. New York. 194 p.

Woodger, Joseph H. — 1952. *Biology and Language: An Introduction to the Methodology of the Biological Sciences, Including Medicine.* Cambridge Univ. Press. England. 364 p.

P

Brenner, Charles — 1955. *An Elementary Textbook of Psychoanalysis.* Int'l. Univ. Press. New York. 219 p.

Colby, Kenneth M. — 1955. *Energy and Structure in Psychoanalysis.* Ronald Press. New York. 154 p.

Dostoyevsky, Fyodor — 1960. *The Idiot* Translated by D. Magarshack. Penguin Books Ltd., Harmondsworth, Middlesex, England.

Erikson, Erik H. — 1964. *Insight and Responsibility.* 2nd Ed. W. W. Norton. New York. 445 p.

Fenichel, Otto — 1945. *The Psychoanalytic Theory of Neurosis.* W. W. Norton. New York. 2nd Vol.

Ferenczi, Sandor — 1926. *Further Contributions to the Theory and Technique of Psycho-analysis.* L. & Virginia Woolf at the Hogarth Press and the Inst. of Psycho-analysis. London. 473 p.

Freud, Anna — 1946. *The Ego and the Mechanisms of Defence.* Translated by C. Baines. Int'l. Univ. Press. New York. 196 p.

Freud, Sigmund — 1936. *The Problem of Anxiety.* Translated by H. A. Bunker. The Psychoanalytic Quarterly Press and W. W. Norton. New York. 165 p.

———— 1959. *Collected Papers.* Basic Books. New York.

Groddeck, Georg Walther — 1950. *The Book of the It.* Funk & Wagnalls. New York.

152

*Categorized
Bibliography*

P

Kubie, Lawrence S.

1950. *Practical and Theoretical Aspects of Psychoanalysis.* Int'l. Univ. Press, New York. Revised 1960. Praeger Paperbacks. New York. 258 p.

Lewin, Bertram.

1950. *The Psychoanalysis of Elation.* W. W. Norton. New York.

Rapaport, David

1960. *Structure of Psychoanalytic Theory.* Int'l. Univ. Press. New York.

Spitz, Rene A.

1965. *The First Year of Life.* Int'l. Univ. Press, New York.

Waelder, Robert

1960. *Basic Theory of Psychoanalysis.* Int'l. Univ. Press, New York. 273 p.

————

1962. "Psychoanalysis, Scientific Method and Philosophy." J. Am. Psychoanalytic Assn. *X:* 617-637.

Farley, B. G.
W. A. Clark

1954. "Simulation of Self-Organizing Systems by Digital Computer." IRE Trans. PGI 1-4: 78-84.

————

1960. "Activity in Networks of Neuron-like Elements." 4th London Symposium on Information Theory.

Braun, Edward L.

1963. *Digital Computer Design Logic, Circuitry and Synthesis.* Academic Press. New York and London.

Gabor, D.
W. Wilby
R. Woodcock

1961. "A Universal Nonlinear Filter Predictor and Simulator Which Optimizes Itself by a Learning Process." Proc. Inst. Elec. Engrs. *108:* Part B.

Hawkins, J. K.

1961. "Self-Organizing Systems — A Review and Commentary." Proc. IRE Jan.: 31-48.

Uttley, A. M.

1956. "Conditional Probability Machines and Conditioned Reflexes" in *Automata Studies.* Princeton Univ. Press, Princeton, New Jersey. pp. 253-275.

Wiener, N.

1948. "Time, Communication, and the Nervous System." Ann. N. Y. Acad. Sci. *50* (4): 197.

O

Bartlett, Sir Frederic C

1958. *Thinking: An Experimental and Social Study.* Basic Books. New York. 203 p.

Boring, Edwin G.

1953. "A History of Introspection." Psychol. Bull. *50:* 169-189.

Bruner, Jerome S.
C. C. Goodman

1947. "Value and Need as Organizing Factors in Perception." J. Abn. Soc. Psychol. *42.*

Bruner, Jerome S.
Goodnow, Jacqueline J.
Austin, George A.

1956. *A Study of Thinking.* Wiley & Sons. New York. 330 p.

Categorized
Bibliography

O

Grinker, Roy R. Helen MacGill Hughes (eds.).   1956. *Toward a Unified Theory of Human Behavior.* Basic Books. New York. 375 p.

Hebb, D. O.   1949. *The Organization of Behavior: A Neuropsychological Theory.* Wiley & Sons. New York. 335 p.

Hilgard, Ernest R.   1956. *Theories of Learning.* Appleton-Century-Crofts. New York.

Hooker, Davenport   1952. *The Prenatal Origin of Behavior.* Univ. of Kansas Press, Lawrence, Kansas. 143 p.

Hull, Clark L.   1933. *Hypnosis and Suggestibility, An Experimental Approach.* Appleton-Century. New York and London. 416 p.

James, William   1929. *The Varieties of Religious Experience: A Study in Human Nature.* Longmans, Green; New York - London, Bombay - Calcutta.

————   1950. *The Principles of Psychology.* Dover Publications. New York. 2 Vols. in 1.

Klüver, Heinrich   1966. *Mescaline and Mechanism of Hallucinations.* Univ. of Chicago Press, Chicago, Ill.

Lewin, Kurt   1936. *Principles of Topological Psychology.* McGraw-Hill. New York - London.

Luria, Alexandr R.   1961. *The Role of Speech in the Regulation of Normal and Abnormal Behavior.* Pergamon Press. New York. 100 p.

Pavlov, I. P.   1957. *Experimental Psychology and Other Essays.* Philosophical Library. New York.

Piaget, Jean   (1932-1952) 1959. *The Language and Thought of the Child.* Translated by Marjorie Gabain. 3rd E. Rev. Harcourt Brace, New York; Kegan Paul, Trench, Trubner, London; Humanities, New York. 251 p.

————   1954. *The Construction of Reality in the Child.* Basic Books. New York.

————   1953-1956. *The Origin of Intelligence in the Child.* Routledge & Paul. London, 1956 Int'l. Univ. Press, New York. 425 p.

————   1962. *Play, Dreams and Imitation in Children.* W. W. Norton. New York.

Skinner, B. F.   1957. *Verbal Behavior.* Appleton. New York.

Stevens, Stanley S. (ed.)   1951. *Handbook of Experimental Psychology.* Wiley & Sons. New York.

154

Categorized
Bibliography

Vygotskii, Lev S.

O

1962. *Thought and Language*. Ed. and translated by E. Haufmann and G. Vakar. M.I.T. Press, Cambridge, Mass. 168 p.

I

Abramson, H. A.

1955. "Lysergic Acid Diethylamide (LSD-25): III. As An Adjunct to Psychotherapy with Elimination of Fear of Homosexuality." J. Psychol. *39*: 127.

Abramson, H. A. (ed.)

1967. *The Use of LSD-25 in Psychotherapy and Alcoholism*. The Bobbs-Merrill Co., Inc., Indianapolis, New York, Kansas City. 697 p.

————

1939. *Association for Research in Nervous and Mental Disease*. The Inter-relationship of Mind and Body. (Assoc. Proc. 1938). Williams & Wilkins. Baltimore, Maryland. 381 p.

————

1952. Association for Research in Nervous and Mental Disease. *Patterns of Organization in the Central Nervous System*. (Assoc. Proc. 1950). Williams & Wilkins. Baltimore, Maryland. 581 p.

————

1954. Association for Research in Nervous and Mental Disease. *Genetics and the Inheritance of Integrated Neurological and Psychiatric Patterns*. (Assoc. Proc. 1953). Williams & Wilkins, Baltimore, Maryland. 425 p.

Cohen, Sidney

1965. *The Beyond Within: The LSD Story*. Atheneum, New York.

Dobshansky, Theodosius G.

1955. *Evolution, Genetics and Man*. Wiley & Sons. New York. 398 p.

Elkes, Joel

1963. *Subjective and Objective Observations in Psychiatry*. (The Harvey Lectures, Series 57.) Academic Press. New York.

Holzinger, R.

1964. "Analytic and Integrative Therapy with the LSD-25." J. Existential Psychiat. *4*: 225-236.

Kubie, Lawrence

1945. "The Therapeutic Role of Drugs in the Process of Repression, Dissociation and Synthesis." Psychosomatic Med. 7: 147-151.

Leuner, H.

1962. *Die Experimentelle Psychose*. Springer Verlag. Berlin.

Ling, T. M.
J. Buckman

1963. *Lysergic Acid (LSD-25) and Ritalin in the Treatment of Neurosis*. Lambarde Press. London.

Categorized
Bibliography

I

Pahnke, Walter N.　1967. "The Contribution of the Psychology of Religion to the Therapeutic Use of the Psychedelic Substances." Chapt. 7 in *The Use of LSD-25 in Psychotherapy and Alcoholism.* H. A. Abramson (ed.) pp. 629-649. The Bobbs-Merrill Co., Inc., Indianapolis, New York, Kansas City.

Ruesch, Jurgen
Gregory Bateson　1951. *Comminication, The Social Matrix of Psychiatry.* Norton. New York. 314 p.

Sandison, R. A.
A. M. Spencer
J. D. Whitelaw　1954. "The Therapeutic Value of Lysergic Acid Diethylamide in Mental Illness." J. Mentl. Sci. *100:* 491-507.

Sandison, R. A.　1955. "LSD Treatment for Psychoneurosis. Lysergic Acid Diethylamide for Release of Repression." Nurs. Mirror (London) *100:* 1529.

Savage, Charles　1956. "The LSD Psychosis as a Transaction Between the Psychiatrist and Patient." In *Lysergic Acid Diethylamide and Mescaline in Experimental Psychiatry.* L. Cholden (ed.). Grune & Stratton, New York. p.35

Sherwood, J. N.
M. J. Stolaroff
W. W. Harmon　1962. "The Psychedelic Experience — a New Concept in Psychotherapy." J. Neuropsychiat. *3:* 370-375.

Szaz, Thomas S.　1961. *The Myth of Mental Illness: Foundations of a Theory of Personal Conduct.* Hoeber-Harper. New York. 337 p.

Unger, Sanford M.　1964. "LSD and Psychotherapy: a Bibliography of the English Language Literature." The Psychedelic Review *I* (4): 442-449.

H

Bernheim, H.　1888. *Hypnosis and Suggestion in Psychotherapy.* "A Treatise on the Nature and Uses of Hypnotism." Translated from the 2nd revised ed. by C. A. Herter. 1964. University Books, New Hyde Park, N. Y. 428 p.

Clark, John Howard　1967. "The Structure of Hypnotic Procedure." 5th International Congress on Cybernetics. 11-15 Sept. 1967. Namur, Bruxelles, Belgium.

Hull, Clark L.　1933. *Hypnosis and Suggestibility.* "An Experimental Approach." The Century Psychology Series, R. M. Elliott (ed.). D. Appleton-Century Co., Inc., New York, London. 416 p.

Categorized
Bibliography

H

Gill, Merton M.
Margaret Brenman

1961. *Hypnosis and Related States.* Psychoanalytic Studies in Regression. International Universities Press, Inc. New York. 405 p.

Lasker, Eric G.

1967. "Computerized Induction of Hypnosis." 5th International Congress on Cybernetics. 11-15 Sept. 1967. Namur, Bruxelles, Belgium.

AUTHOR'S PAPERS

Lilly, J. C.

1956. "Mental Effects of Reduction of Ordinary Levels of Physical Stimuli on Intact, Healthy Persons." In *Psychiat. Res. Report 5.* American Psychiatric Assn. Washington, D. C. 1-9 pp.

————

1958. "Some Considerations Regarding Basic Mechanisms of Positive and Negative Types of Motivations." Am. J. Psychiat. *115:* 498-504.

————

1957. "Stop and Start Systems" in *Neuropharmacology.* Transactions of the Fourth Conference, Josiah Macy, Jr. Foundation. Princeton, N. J. pp. 153-179.

————

1958. "Rewarding and Punishing Systems in the Brain" in *The Central Nervous System and Behavior.* Transactions of the First Conference, Josiah Macy Jr. Foundation. Princeton, N. J. p. 247.

————

1959. "Stop and Start Effects" in *The Central Nervous System and Behavior.* Transactions of the Second Conference, Josiah Macy Jr. Foundation and National Science Foundation. Princeton, N. J. pp. 56-112.

————

1962. "The Effect of Sensory Deprivation on Consciousness" in *Man's Dependence on the Earthly Atmosphere.* K. E. Schaefer (ed.). Proceedings 1st Int'l. Symp. on Submarine and Space Medicine. New London, Conn. 1958. Macmillan Co. New York. pp. 93-95.

Lilly, J. C.
J. T. Shurley

1961. "Experiments in Solitude, in Maximum Achievable Physical Isolation with Water Suspension, of Intact Healthy Persons." (Symposium, USAF Aerospace Medical Center, San An-

*Categorized
Bibliography*

AUTHOR'S PAPERS

tonio, Texas, 1960, in *Psychophysiological* As-
pects of Space Flight. Columbia Univ. Press.
New York. pp. 238-247.

Lilly, J. C.
1961. "The Biological Versus Psychoanalytic Dichotomy." Bull. of Phila. Assoc. for Psychoanal.
11: 116-119.

——————
1963. "Critical Brain Size and Language." Perspec-
tives in Biol. & Med. *6*: 246-255.

——————
1965. "Vocal Mimicry in *Tursiops*: Ability to
Match Numbers and Durations of Human Vocal
Bursts." Science *147*: 300-301.

——————
1966. "Communication with Extraterrestrial Intelligence." (1965 IEEE Military Electronics Conf.
Washington, D. C. Sept. 1965.) IEEE Spectrum
3 (3): 159-160.

——————
1967. *The Mind of the Dolphin: A Nonhuman
Intelligence*. Doubleday & Company, Inc. Garden
City, New York. 331 p.

Lilly, J. C.
Alice M. Miller
1968. "Reprogramming the Sonic Output of the
Dolphin: Sonic Burst-Count Matching." JASA
43: 1412-1424.

◻ Abstract

Programming and Metaprogramming in The Human Biocomputer (Effects of Psychedelic Substances)

The basic assumptions on which we operate are as follows. Each mammalian brain functions as a computer, with properties, programs, and metaprograms partly to be defined and partly to be determined by observation. The human computer contains at least 13 billion active elements and hence is functionally and structurally larger than any artificially built computer of the present era. This human computer has the properties of modern artificial computers of large size, plus additional ones not yet achieved in the non-biological machines. This human computer has stored-program properties, and stored-metaprogram properties as well. Among other known properties are self-programming and self-metaprogramming. Programming codes and metaprogramming language are different for each human, depending upon the developmental, experimental, genetic, educational, accidental and self-chosen, variables, elements and values. Basically, the verbal forms are those of the native language of the individual, modulated by non-verbal language elements acquired in the same epochs of his development.

Each such computer has scales of self-measuration and self-evaluation. Constant and continuous computations are being done, giving aim and goal distance estimates of external reality performances and internal reality achievements.

Comparison scales are now set up between human computers for performance measures of each and of several in concert. Each computer models other computers of importance to itself, beginning immediately *post partum,* with greater or lesser degrees of error.

The phenomemon computer interlock facilities model instruction and operation. One computer interlocks with one or more other computers above and below the level of awareness any time the communicational distance is sufficiently small to bring the interlock functions above threshold level.

In the complete physical absence of other external computers within the critical interlock distance, the self-directed and other-directed programs can be clearly detected, analyzed, recomputed, and reprogrammed, and new metaprograms initiated by the solitudinous computer itself. In this physical reality (which is as completely attenuated as possible environment with solitude), maximum intensity, maximum complexity, and maximum speed of reprogramming are achievable by the self.

In the field of scientific research, such a computer can function in many different ways—from the pure, austere thought processes of theory and mathematics to the almost random data absorption of the naturalistic approach with newly-found systems, or to the coordinated interlock with other human computers of an engineering effort.

At least two extreme major techniques of data-collection analysis exist for individual scientists: (1) artificially created, controlled-element, invented, devised-system methods; and (2) methods involving the participant-observer, who interacts intimately and experientially with naturally given elements, with non-human or human computers as parts of the system.

The former is the current basis of individual physical-chemical research; the latter is one basis for individual explorative, first-discovery research of organisms having brains larger than those of humans.

Sets of human motivational procedural postulates for the interlock research method on non-human beings, with computers as large as and larger than the human computers, are sought. Some of these methods involve the establishment of long periods—perhaps months or years—of human to other organism computer interlock. It is hoped that this interlock will be of a quality and value sufficiently high to permit interspecies communication efforts on both sides on an intense, highly structured level.

The chemical agent lysergic acid di-ethylamide (LSD-25) has been shown by many investigators to cause large changes in the modes of functioning of the human biocomputer. The dosage to obtain various effects ranges from 25 to 1000 micrograms per subject per session. The detectable primary effects have a time course, a latency of 20-40 minutes, from time of administration and endure for 4 to 12 hours for single or divided doses, with a peak effect at 2 to 3 hours. At the same dose level, such effects cannot be repeated for 72 to 144 hours. Detectable secondary and tertiary effects have a longer time course. With sufficiently sensitive testing techniques, secondary effects with half-life of 1 week to 6 weeks have been described. Tertiary effects can be detected for 1 to 2 years.

The descriptions in the literature of the primary effects vary considerably. The frameworks of these descriptions show a great variety of phenomenological, philosophical, medical, psychiatric, psychological, social and religious conceptualizations. Published mechanisms and models of the phenomena are found to be unsatisfactory. Published experiments resulting from the use of these models are also not satisfactory.

As a result of this dissatisfaction with published materials, a new model was constructed: the human biocomputer. Interactive experiments were designed to test this model with LSD-25 sessions. The subject was pre-programmed with the general concepts of the model over several months before the first session, and with specific programs to be tested 12 hours to one hour before each session. During separate sessions (100-400 micro-grams dose range), programming was done (a) by self, (b) written instruc-tions, (c) taped instructions, (d) environmental control and (e) one other person. Results were dictated during some sessions or transcribed immedi-ately after each session; follow-up analyses were similarly recorded for periods up to several months.

Modifications of the model were made as the necessity arose during the long-term analyses, and introduced in each later session as specific instructions. The model is one that continues to evolve in as general purpose and open-ended a way as is possible for this investigator.

This account gives a report of the current state of this model of the human biocomputer, some of the properties found, the programming and metaprogramming done, the concepts evolved, the special isolation-solitude environment, and special metaprogramming techniques developed.

Communication Research Institute
Scientific Report No. CR10167